Carb Cycling

How to Lose Weight, Shed Fat, and Live a Healthier Life Without Giving Up On Your Favorite Meals

by Alice Redfield

Table of contents

INTRODUCTION

With many studies conducted on this topic, and lingering debates surrounding the notion of carbohydrate intake, this book is intended to delve deeply into how cycling carb intake carries many benefits for reducing fat percentage, specifically. While cutting down the percentage of fat on your body is subject to many different factors, with some being pre-existing- such as genetics- this text will explain how cycling carb intake is the most reliable and consistent methods of reducing one's overall body fat.

Granted, starting a new diet is a very challenging process and carries many obstacles mentally, physically, and even emotionally. However, by systematically approaching your diet, with careful consideration given to how your body is responding to the new changes that you are implementing, you will be well on your way to enjoying all of the inherent benefits that carb cycling has to offer you.

While there are certainly numerous benefits associated with your intake of carbs, it is integral to note that more medical research still needs to be done in order to unveil all of the effects and potential benefits associated with this process. Given the number of studies of dependable studies that have already been conducted, along with the plethora personal testimonies and anecdotes from dependable sources, you do not have to worry much about how this diet will affect you. The need for more research is merely a manner through which more information can be uncovered pertaining to cycling one's carb consumption. This will provide you with a much deeper understanding of the specific ways that this diet will influence your body and help you reach your desired goals.

Everyone is different in both body and lifestyle. The great thing about carb cycling is there is more than one way to incorporate it into your lifestyle. There are different levels of intensity which determine how quickly you experience results. You can include reward meals and cheat days into carb cycling if you plan them properly.

No matter what cycle you choose you still follow the same number of meals, grams of fat/protein and carb goals. The only thing that will change is the carbs you choose if you are having a cheat meal or a cheat day. You still eat all the vegetables and your fruit. In other words, the foundation of carb cycling doesn't change.

Thanks for downloading this book. It's my firm belief that it will provide you with all the answers to your questions.

History

There was a time in the 1970s and 1980s called the 'high-carb mania.' Most of the popular diets of that time encouraged the intake of large amounts of carbohydrates. However, this perception changed drastically in the 1990s, and an exact opposite became popular. The diets of the 1990s, and later, concentrated on reducing the carbohydrate in the diet, giving rise to the 'low-carb mania.'

With that said, people are still unclear about how the carbs are used up in the human body. More precisely, the contribution of carb amounts to any weight loss program needs to be understood. Without any understatement, it can be said that your carb intake can be the game changer in your weight loss program and be responsible for weight loss. On the other hand, it might just be the macronutrient that can destroy your plan completely.

Today, the scenario has changed, and there are a plethora of resources available for people to study and know what their bodies are going through, with and without a weight loss regime. Despite this availability of resources, people are still facing weight issues so much so that obesity is one of the most common problems faced by the world today. This brings us to question as to why the scenario is deteriorating.

After much contemplation, experts have stated that the reason behind the increasing problem of obesity is that none of the existing fitness systems understands the functioning of the human body. Most of the existing dietary approaches end up lowering the body's metabolism. As a result, the body loses all its energy and motivation to lose weight, putting the weight loss program on a complete halt. Evidently, putting the body on a constant amount of carbohydrates cannot solve the issues, and you'll need to vary the carbs in your diet to keep the ball rolling as far as weight loss is concerned.

Franco Carlotto created carb cycle regiment in the 1990s, in his attempt to prepare for the Mr. World Fitness Title. In the process, he also helped millions of people around the world in maintaining a lean and healthy body. The main objective of this dietary approach was to help people achieve not just their long-term weight loss goals but to reach both the short-term and long-term milestones in time.

This technique has been developed from the analysis of how our ancestors ate and depleted their carb storage to maintain a healthy body. Although the times have changed, the human body and the way it functions remains the same. Therefore, the solution to weight loss issues also remains the same in the 21st century. We have to understand and manipulate our own carb storage system to get the weight loss results we expect.

The carb cycle approach requires an individual to alternate high carb and low carb cycles on a daily basis, regulating the natural storage system of the body in such a way that the body doesn't store anything and burns more than what is expected on a daily and weekly basis. The low carb days deplete the body of its carbohydrates. However, the high carb days replenish the carb reserves. In this way, the body doesn't get exhausted of its energy and resources at any time. On a personal level, you don't have to give up on all your carbohydrate-rich foods altogether. You can just vary them on the basis of the day of the cycle and still reach your weight loss milestones.

Most practitioners of carb cycling recommend a basic carb cycling for beginners giving them a slow start an introduction to the world of dietary approaches. One of the best things about this dietary approach is that it doesn't restrict the individual to a point where he or she will start cheating on the diet. Therefore, the guilt that most people feel from not being able to follow the regime properly, and losing the motivation doesn't have much of an effect on people following a carb cycling approach.

Any carb cycling approach is not just a dietary plan, but it is a complete way of life. It is a comprehensive fitness guide for an individual to follow throughout their lives. The scope for adjustment in the carb cycling approach allows people to alter it on the basis of the changing needs of their body. Therefore, they can carry on with this fitness regime regardless of the age and fitness levels they reach. Although carb cycling is a relatively new approach to dieting, its popularity speaks volumes about its effectiveness for people across ages and gender.

Getting Started with Carb Cycling

Carb cycling can be performed in many different ways. In fact, an individual performing carb cycling can vary the high carb and low carb cycles in several unique ways. The beauty of this dietary approach is that it can take a lot of fine-tuning and adjustments as you move forward with it.

Although the first level of variation is performed when you decide the training sessions and cycles of carb days that you plan to follow, many higher-level adjustments at the week-level can also be performed. For instance, you can go on a low carb diet for the first 11 days and take a high carb break for 3 days that follow (12th, 13th, and 14th day).

Besides this, you can also experiment with the number of calories you consume on a daily basis, keeping the weekly limit intact. On a higher level, you may also change the weekly limit to see the level at which you can stretch your body to push itself for weight loss. On the basis of your goals, exercise routine, and lifestyle, you can chalk out a plan for yourself to get started.

You need to understand at this stage that your tolerance levels, activity, and muscle mass will determine the right amount of carbs per day for you. Therefore, there is no perfect formula to determine this. You will need to experiment with the carb values to see which value works the best for you. You may choose a daily-changing or monthly-changing carb cycling approach depending on your body type and activity level. For instance, an individual who has average activity levels can do just fine with a monthly approach, while an athlete will require daily changes in carb cycling.

Carbohydrate Food Sources Recommended For You

Foods rich in fructose must be avoided at all costs. With that said, there is a long list of foods that can be included in your diet. As a rule, it is good to include foods that are rich in minerals, vitamins, and fiber. A word of caution here is that you must not treat high carb days as opportunities to splurge on all the high-calorie desserts and ruin all of your efforts. Therefore, making healthier choices is extremely important. Some of the foods that can easily be added to your diet include:

- Whole Grains

Grains that have not been modified are known to have several health benefits, apart from being a perfect inclusion for your carb cycling diet plan. Some useful sources of whole grains include oats, rice, and quinoa.

- Vegetables

The mineral and vitamin content associated with each vegetable is different. Moreover, the color balance is given by the inclusion of different vegetables also adds color high nutritive value to the food.

- Unprocessed Fruits

As is the case with vegetables, fruits also have different abilities and benefits. For instance, berries have anti-oxidant benefits without putting any glycemic load on the body.

- Legumes

It is always a good idea to include carbohydrates that take longer to digest because they reduce hunger and curb cravings. In addition, foods that are rich in fiber and minerals are also beneficial. A food type that includes the benefits of both of these types of foods is a legume.

- Tubers

One of the richest sources of carbohydrates are tubers like sweet potatoes and potatoes. When on a high carb day, it is a good idea to pick them for a quick increase in carbs.

Creating a Meal Plan for Carb Cycling

Although carb cycling is a good middle path as it does not restrict your carb intake completely and it lets you take a few high carb dishes, it doesn't mean that you can feast on pasta every alternate day. Moreover, carb cycling is recommended not just for people who are willing to lose weight; it is a recommended dietary strategy for people who are willing to build muscle.

One of the fundamental things about eating healthy carbs every now and then is that it keeps your metabolism steady. Moreover, the addition of vegetables and proteins to your regular diet in proportionate quantities keeps the insulin levels low enough so as to ensure that you lose weight and not lose muscle.

Carb cycling can be changed and altered to fit into your routine. However, if you are still unsure about where to start, here are a few things that you can consider and implement for putting together a weekly carb cycling menu.

- Identify the Right Formula

The ideal plan for carb cycling is to alternate high carb and low carb days for the six days of the week and reserve reward meals for the seventh day. With that said, you may have different health objectives and personal health. Therefore, you will need to alter the carb cycling menu according to these factors. For example, if you wish to lose weight, you can be on five low carb days and follow it with two high carb days.

On the contrary, if you wish to add weight and build muscle mass, you can have around five high carb days and follow them with two low carb days. However, if you put yourself on this regime, remember not to put all the high carb days together. In fact, alternate them with low carb days and space out all kinds of days across the landscape of the week.

- Choose Your Foods Wisely

The carb cycling approach may sound to many as if it is okay to be on meat for the low carb days and indulge in your favorite pasta for the rest of the week. This is not true at all. When you are on a high carb day, you can derive a majority of the calories from whole grains like legumes and fruits. They will play an instrumental role in keeping your energy levels high without letting you compromise on your weight loss goals.

The low carbs days are usually the toughest to decide on meals. Therefore, it is recommended that you derive your protein intake from eggs, tofu, and lean meats during this period. You can choose any vegetable to complement the protein. Try to distance yourself from processed foods and keep your grocery shopping restricted to fresh staples.

• Eat the Right Snacks

The idea behind carb cycling is not to starve and yet help you lose weight at the same time. It gives you the leverage to indulge in small snacks every now and then. If a bowl of sugary snack can help you remain on track, you are allowed to have it. The only condition is that you must have it on a high carb day.

• Make a Meal Plan

Now that you have planned all the proteins and grains that you need to include in your diet, the next thing is to create a daily menu to follow. The typical calorie intake for men should be around 1500 calories a day while the same for a woman should not exceed 1200 calories.

Keeping this in view, it is also equally important to remember that this value varies from individual to individual. It is good to maintain this calorie count on a daily basis. Moreover, it is equally important to maintain the macronutrient constitution of the food you eat.

You can contact a dietician or use any of online calculators available to count the macronutrient constitution required per body weight to lose weight or gain mass. Another piece of advice for you is that you must eat your breakfast as early as possible after waking up. The rest of the allocated calories for the day can be spread out to four to six comparatively smaller meals.

Typical Meal Plans

A day can be divided into five meals: breakfast, morning snack, lunch, evening snack, and dinner. For a low carb day, you can have 2 eggs for breakfast; a berry protein shakes for the morning snack and oatmeal for the evening snack. The lunch can include grilled chicken with asparagus while the dinner can be steak with vegetables.

On the other hand, on a high carb day, oatmeal with fruits can be your breakfast, followed by fruit like apples along with almond butter or honey as a morning snack. A turkey sandwich or burger for lunch and salad for the evening snack will make a good high carb combination. Your high carb day can end with grilled chicken and pasta.

On the basis of your personal preferences and availability of ingredients, you can pick and try all of the recipes.

How Does Carb Cycling

Work?

Carb cycling, also known as carbohydrate cycling, is a weight management technique that requires certain meal plans to be incorporated with regulated types of food groups in them. Usually, the food items included in the meal plans are monitored for carbohydrate content. As the name of the diet program implies, carbohydrate-laden food items are important to monitor because they determine the type of food item that will be eaten for each meal on any given day.

There are different aspects to the carbohydrate cycle that you should understand.

You should keep in mind that there are six meals that you have to consume each day. Each of the meals eaten should have regular intervals between each other. This will help to ensure that you develop a regular and highly functional metabolic rate for your digestive system.

During a high carb-laden day, you are allowed to consume as many carbohydrates as you want, but only for certain meals within the day.

Out of the six meals that you will eat on that day, you may consume as many carbs as you desire for four of the meals. You may eat carbs as soon as you have consumed the recommended amount of fats and proteins.

Aside from your unlimited carbohydrate consumption, you must eat a piece of fruit with 50 to 100 calories before you consume any carbs. The fruit you consume contains fructose that will help your body to produce more energy. The body can produce more energy by virtue of glycogen storage inside your liver. Even if fructose is a form of sugar, this cannot affect the fat production in your body because the consumption of 50 to 100 calories is not enough to elicit an effect in your body. Instead, the fructose value that you consume can help promote prolonged satiety for your digestive system. Thus, you will have a decreased need to eat additional meals in between the predetermined six meals on this specific day. And, this will prevent you from overeating.

The Low- carbs day may be considered as the most complicated among the three phases of this diet program due to certain macronutrient goals that you must fulfill.

For this specific carb cycling day, you must consume carbohydrates for only three out of the six meals that you eat. Before you consume any carbohydrates, you need to include the prescribed amount of protein and fat in your diet. Moreover, you must consume a small fruit with 50 to 100 calories in it beforehand.

The recommended amount of carbohydrates is set at one gram of carbs for every one pound of weight in your body each day. After computing for the total value of carbs that you must consume each day, you would then divide this value by three. This is the amount of carbs that you are allowed to eat for three out of the six meals during your low carbs day. You should note that the amount of carbs that you need to consume for each meal should be equally distributed in order to ensure consistency in your metabolic rate.

A no-carbs day is considered the easiest, but most important, among the phases of carb cycling.

The no-carbs day is regarded as the most controversial part of the carbs cycling diet program. As the term suggests, you are not allowed to eat any food items with carbs for the six meals that you will have for that day. But, you still need to consume the minimum amount of fat and protein for all your meals to prevent delaying your muscle development process. Apart from these instructions, you may consume as much protein as you want for your meals on this day.

Initially, you may find it difficult to get through this day. One way to keep on track is to motivate yourself by thinking about the high carbs day that lies only a few days ahead.

There are numerous factors which can determine if you will emerge successful while engaging in the carbs cycling diet program.

You are able to control some of these factors of the diet program. But, you cannot manipulate the other factors of this diet because they are fixed and based on the specific genetic aspects of your body.

If you want to build a solid foundation in order to ensure success for your diet program, setting certain diet-related goals can help you do this.

Your goals will determine the success rate that you will attain at the end of the diet program, once you complete the program. Experts recommend that you adhere to a set time, as well as realistic, objective, specific, and concrete goals. Composing your goals in this manner will help you to stay motivated. These goals will help you to assess your progress during the time you are on a diet.

Before you start off with the actual diet program, you should set your long term and short term goals. In the process of goal setting, you should already know what you want to attain after the program. In the long run, this will tell you how much satisfaction you will attain after reaching your goals.

Body builds are uncontrollable variables that can somehow determine your success rate in the carb cycling diet program.

Different body types have different reactions to certain diet programs that are introduced. Therefore, you must have your body type assessed in order to determine how you use the program to create significant and positive results for your body.

Ectomorphic is known as the thin body type. People with this body type have a small and rather delicate body frame and bone structure. Experts do not usually recommend this diet program for people with ectomorphic body types because they already have high metabolic rates used to get rid of the adipose tissues in their body.

Mesomorphic is known as the lean body type. People with this body type have naturally athletic physiques. Given this fact, mesomorphs usually manifest with large muscle groups and sturdy bone structures.

Endomorphic is a soft and solid body type. Compared to the two previous body types presented, the endomorphic body type tends to have the largest proportions of fat. People with this body type are the most sensitive to carbohydrates. This implies that they should consume fewer carbohydrates because they tend to gain more fats compared to the mesomorphs and the ectomorphs. Given these premises, endomorphs have the most weight management benefits if they maximize the intricacies of the program.

Your lifestyle can tell you how successful you will be on this diet program even before you start.

For most diet programs out there, you must also incorporate various workout routines and physical activities into your daily schedule. This activity is important because it will set your major muscle groups to work. As soon as they are set to work, you initiate the processes of fat breakdown and muscle buildup. You must do these things for the rest of your life.

Support systems can mean a lot, especially when you are going through difficult phases of your carb cycle.

Working with a support system can make you accountable for everything that you are about to do, which is related to your diet program. The right support system reminds you to fulfill your goals and plans. They can also affirm and encourage you when you are successful. If you are doing something that can benefit you in the long run, they will let you know. Some support systems can even assist you in creating diet and exercise alternatives.

Like other diet programs out there, the carb cycling diet includes different goals for each phase that you go through while in the cycle.

The main goal of this diet program is to help you lose those unwanted pounds. In the process, carb cycling should help you to develop lean muscle mass instead of wasting muscle mass. As soon as you see that you are getting rid of fats while toning up your body, you will eventually get motivated to continue the program.

Monitoring your progress as you go along the diet program can help you to boost your motivation levels further. To help you monitor your achievements while participating in the program, you have to weigh yourself and take measurements regularly, such as hip to waist ratio and waistline measurements. You must obtain baseline measurements for these aspects as these will serve as the base of comparisons for your next measurements. Afterward, you will need to take measurements every six to eight weeks that you are on a diet. On average, each cycle of this diet program lasts for three to four days.

Because workouts are considered a part of any type of effective diet program, you should make specific considerations when working out while you are involved in the carb cycling diet program.

Right after performing all your workout routines, you will have to consume 30 to 50 grams worth of protein. This will help to reinforce the process of muscle development and assist you in muscle repair. If you are on a low carbs or high carbs day, during the day of the workout, you have to follow up your protein intake with some carbohydrates. If you want to yield better results, you have to consume food items such as whey protein and oatmeal.

THE CARB CYCLE

Carb cycling is something very interesting and adventurous, as there is some science and art – both involved in it. You need to choose a special plan that has been devised by a professional. Tracking progress is also very important to have an idea about the results. It is a good thing that is the plan is not based on starvation techniques, as you cannot afford to slow down your metabolism. When you starve, your metabolism also slows down, and it affects your total muscle mass. Not only this, but your overall health also suffers. Don't think of losing fat by starving. In the first phase of this plan, you will go through the calorie maintenance program.

In the beginning, you will need to reduce calories to some extent. But it is something different from starving yourself. It is all about putting the focus on reducing the calories that you consume after having carbohydrate food items. Our body needs energy and muscles to perform different actions. If you exercise on a regular basis, it is a good thing that your body does make use of muscle mass for fueling your body. It actually makes use of fat to cover the glycogen levels. There are high days and low days in a carb cycle that help in managing the glycogen levels. It actually is a cycle that consists of some ups and downs.

During high days, you focus on refilling glycogen supply in order to get rid of it again within some days. The major benefit of this cycle is that you get a chance of losing fat and retaining muscle mass. You don't push your body to the point of starvation but only focus on burning fat for fuel. Carbohydrates are best for refueling the low level of glycogen in your body. Glycogen is stored in two different places in your system. The liver is the main store where glycogen is stored, and the primary storage is located just close to the surface of our skin. Our body continuously tries to restore the lost glycogen levels.

When there is not enough carbohydrate to be used as a source of fuel, your body will make use of fat storage. When you force your body to starve, it opts to use muscle mass for the process of catabolism. The main reason is that your muscles also have glycogen stored in them. It is actually a very expensive form of calorie that helps in maintaining muscle mass. Understand the cycle that leads to rapid weight loss, which might not be good for you. Starvation leads to slow metabolism, and it results in muscle loss eventually.

When you break muscle, you also lose water and glycogen with it. It leads to rapid loss of weight, and it means that you are consuming very few calories than the standard amount. It is recommended to have carbs on a daily basis, and your diet must include 20% carbs in it. Carbs actually help in retaining muscles mass. When you have enough and essential carbs in your system, your body won't need to make use of the protein. Carbs actually have a sparing effect on the protein that helps in developing and repairing muscle mass. This explains us one thing that no matter how hard you try to gain and retain muscle mass, it's actually all about the carbs. They always come to the rescue and preserve muscle mass.

If you want to build muscle, it is important to consume carbs also, apart from the proteins. To have the best from the carb cycle, it is recommended to develop muscles in order to retain carbs. Your metabolism will remain active if you have the right lean mass. So it depends on you that how you make it easier for your body to lose fat. Now, you are well aware of the role of carbs in your diet and its importance to help lose weight. That is the reason that many professional trainers and nutritionists recommend taking smaller meals throughout the day to keep your metabolism active. A large meal would not have a good effect on your body. When you consume small meals throughout the day, the thermic system remains active. When heat is produced, it helps in burning calories.

The High Carb Days

•	You will need to stimulate insulin response that will deliver nutrients to various muscle cells and help them grow

•	Eat hard to replenish glycogen reserves that help in fueling your muscles

•	Make you feel energized and happy

The Low Carb Days

•	You trick your body to burn fat and promote fat loss

•	Your muscles start developing, as your body becomes more receptive to the insulin.

You allow your body muscles to grow, repair, and maintain.

Principles of Carb Cycling

Truth be told, the concept of carb cycling has been practiced by bodybuilders even before the idea of such diet was formally presented to the public. Bodybuilders would take in lots of carbs while they are bulking up, and then use carb cycling to shed the excess fats. Seeing that it was an effective practice among the bodybuilders, some personal trainers then tested the regimen on non-bodybuilders to see if it would be just as effective. The results are astounding.

Effectiveness – Just the Right Carb Amounts

The carb cycling diet proved to be effective and were gradually introduced to more fitness enthusiasts, particularly to those who frequently hit the gym, as an alternative for low-carb diets and as a complementary diet program for muscle builders. With this diet, the goal is to consume just enough carbohydrates to fuel your body for exercise or training and still burn fats and make progress towards your weight goals.

The Two Phases of Carb Cycling

There are essentially two types of days in a carb cycling diet, the high-carb and low-carb day. During the high-carb days, the body is refilled with carbohydrates to make it more energized to do exercise or training. The glycogen stores which stimulate the muscles are also replenished, so the body will be prepared to do rigorous activities during the day. Meanwhile, during low-carb days, the body is tricked into burning body fats for energy instead of carbohydrates.

The Fat Burning and Muscle Building Mechanism of The Carb Cycling Diet

As the body is being deprived of carbohydrate supply during low-carb days, the body will enter the state of ketosis in order to produce enough energy to fuel your activities. While on ketosis, the body will burn excess fats so it can convert it into energy, making you lose weight in the process. With regards to muscle building, low-carb days trim excess fat from your muscles and help prepare it to absorb carbohydrates during high-carb days.

As the high-carb days arrive, your body will now be replenished of lost nutrients during low-carb days. At this time, the muscles will be ready to absorb as much carbs as it can to make up for its deprivation. By absorbing carbohydrates, your muscles will start growing without making you consume too much food and supplements.

Note that problems with dehydration, weakness, fatigue, hunger pangs, and cravings are also addressed by carb cycling, thanks to the carb refills that occur once or twice a week. During high-carb days, the dieter will be allowed to consume more carbohydrates compared to a typical no- or low-carb day. The carb refill days have three main objectives:

1.   To replenish the glycogen stores (in the muscle and liver) that have been depleted during intense activities or workout sessions.

2.   To normalize the activity of the thyroid and other hormones that the body was deprived of during low-carb days.

3.   To provide a physical and psychological timeout, which makes this diet more bearable compared to other diet programs.

Being able to refill the supply of glycogen in the body allows the dieter to increase his endurance and muscle mass, which would be impossible in a strictly low-carb diet. However, high-carb days can also be risky if not monitored properly. A person might end up gaining more weight during the carb refill if he consumes more carbohydrates than what is needed to replenish the glycogen stores. Therefore, it is crucial to pay attention to the proper duration and timing of carb refill days and make sure to allocate nutrients to keep the body balanced and healthy properly.

How Many Carbohydrates

are Okay to Eat?

Carb cycling gives you the option to be flexible. As a rule, make sure you are consuming at least 50 grams of carbohydrates on your low-carb days. One formula for determining carb consumption is to consume 1 gram of carbohydrates per pound of body mass. (Note that 50 grams may be lower than this amount). Opt for less intense workouts on these low-carb days. This minimal amount creates an opportunity to use up existing body fuels. And you will end up eating more of the proteins that help in building more muscle mass.

Many women feel they have low energy levels on low-carb days. It is all right to feel this way. Your mind might be telling you, "Nothing is working." Carb cycling makes it pretty easy to remain encouraged. Yes, you can have 50 grams of carbohydrates a day, and you can enjoy the occasional high carb day.

You may consume 120-400 grams of carbs on high-carb days. Woohoo! Calculate about 2-3 grams of carbs per pound of body weight. Therefore, if you weigh 120 pounds, your carb intake should be 240-360 grams. Stick to the lower end of that intake at first, then, gradually add more carbs. Start with 100 grams of carbs and move gradually toward the higher end of the scale.

What kinds of carbohydrates...?

While you are carb cycling, you want to consume nutritious foods.

Good foods to eat:

Dairy

- skim milk

- fat-free yogurt

Grains & Starches

- whole grain bread

- whole grain tortillas

- corn

- oatmeal

- whole grain cereals

- popcorn

- barley

- buckwheat

- whole grain pasta

- potatoes

- peas

I am a huge fan of eating fruits!

Fruit

- apples

- apricots

- berries

- bananas

- kiwi

- grapes

- melon

- oranges

- plums

Muscle building requires protein, and meat is one of the best sources of protein. Include the following in your diet:

Meat, Poultry & Fish

- chicken

- turkey breast

- duck breast

- lean beef

- tuna

- salmon

- shrimp

- lobster

- crab

- trout

• lean pork

The Carb Cycling diet requires eating lots of great veggies.

Vegetables

• asparagus

• broccoli

• cabbage

• carrots

• cauliflower

• celery

• cucumber

• eggplant

• lettuce

• green beans

• mushrooms

• onions

- peppers

- snow peas

- spinach

- tomatoes

- zucchini

Okay, this is a long list. Finally, here are some good sources of fat.

Fats

- low-fat mozzarella

- low-fat cheese

- mayonnaise

- almond butter

- peanut butter

- fish oil

- canola oil

- olive oil

Complete 28-Day Meal Plan

Your average Carb Cycling week will look like this:

- High carb days

- Medium carb day

- Low carb days

It can be changed according to individual requirements, but your meal plan will be similar to this one.

You'll be consuming the two types of meal plans:

1) Protein and carbs

2) Protein and fat

You'll consume protein with fat at low-carb days. Try to eliminate all fats on high-carb days. The protein consumption remains the same on all days. Look for different food sources, but stick to these proportions.

Many people struggle with the calorie count. Here is a good way to figure out the correct size portion to maintain the appropriate calorie count:

Use your fist to calculate portion sizes – fist-size meat and vegetable portions, or a handful of berries, for example.

Understanding Your Body

Food is necessary for everyone. Food is a necessity for the sustenance of life. All the nutrients that sustain the body come from food. Without food, the body dies. A lack of food and the body becomes weak.

On the other side of the scale, too much food intake also makes the body weak. Too much or lack of it can cause many ailments to the body's different organs. Both can contribute to the organs working harder than they normally should. The body is a very efficient machine with different parts that work together. Each organ or part has a unique role to play for the normal operation of the whole body.

Like any machine, fuel is needed to keep the machine running. Food is the fuel for the body. But unlike ordinary fuel, the body needs a more complex form of fuel with different mixtures of nutrients that the different parts or organs require to operate normally.

What is the Right Diet?

The three basic food groups that are good sources of nutrients needed by the body are carbohydrates, protein, and fats. A well-balanced diet must contain all three. Take away any one or more of them, and the result is an imbalanced diet, which is not a good approach for achieving weight loss. Too much is sacrificed for an objective that contributes nothing to the overall health condition.

It's best to follow the basic rule: eat the right amount of food based on how active you are. The more active a person is, the more nutrients are needed. A less active person does not need as much fuel. Excess food will just be stored within the body in the form of blood sugar and cholesterol. Two elements that may have important contributions to the body's sustenance, but in excess can have bad effects.

47

Body Conditioning – Physical or Mental?

A number of factors influence the amount of one's activity: a person's lifestyle, work, and environment. These three are also the main elements in a person's social and economic life. A person's career may not require too much physical activity but more mental activity, or vice versa. Engaging in an activity, either physical or mental, is almost the same. They can both be stressful and energy draining. Both require a good amount of food to restore all the energy that is used.

This is where another complication arises. How much food does one need if the person is more physically active? If the person is more mentally active, what is the right amount of food that one needs to consume?

In the end, every person is different and requires a different amount of energy to meet their needs. Experiment with your diet until you reach a point where you're neither gaining nor losing weight. At this level, your energy levels are being perfectly met.

Whether one is engaged more in mental or in physical activity, that inherent need for nutrients can be satisfied with a proven food intake management method called the carb cycling diet.

The Different Methods of a Carb Cycling Program

Carb cycling is a relatively easy method of controlling or managing body weight by deliberately and methodically scheduling different amounts of carbohydrate intake while maintaining the required amount of protein in the diet. While this dietary program may seem or looks complicated, it's actually quite simple to follow.

A carb cycling diet maintains the required level of nutrients in the body, albeit, on a controlled approach. Whatever nutrition the body needs, the body gets.

The general idea of carb cycling is carbohydrate intake management. Other food groups such as protein and fat are also an essential part of the diet, with protein intake playing an important role in the dietary program.

Deeply Rooted from Bodybuilding

While protein is not really the focus of the diet, it is an essential part of the diet. The right amount of protein needed by the body is maintained at all times of the dietary plan. This is understandable since protein is an essential nutrient for athletes like bodybuilding enthusiasts. The rigors of their training exercises demand a substantial amount of protein. Protein works to maintain and grow muscle, as well as keeps you feeling full.

How About Non-Athletes?

Not everyone has the same protein requirement as athletes. Sedentary people, or those that engage in less physical activity than athletes, require less protein. Heavy physical activities increase amino acid oxidation, thus increasing the need for more protein.

Protein requirements of the body depend on a lot of factors, including a person's age, body weight, and composition, physical activity level, energy reserves, and the intake of carbohydrates.

All About Protein

Protein is the basic element of life itself. It is found everywhere: in every muscle, organ, and gland of the body. Amino acids are the major component of protein. It's what the body needs to heal and maintain itself. Body development and growth also depend on this substance.

When proteins break down during digestion, their amino acid content is not dissolved and absorbed by the body; rather, it's used for other functions of the body. The body does not produce its own amino acids; they are supplied through the food eaten, like meat or nuts or even milk.

Meats are not the only source of protein; they can also be obtained from fish and many dairy products. There are plants that are also rich in protein like soybeans, legumes, and some grains. So there is no need to source all the protein requirement of the body from meat. Some meat, especially red meat contains a high level of fats, which may also contribute to a high level of cholesterol if taken indiscriminately. As much as possible, get your protein intake requirement from lean meat, such as fish and chicken, or plant-based foods, such as soy and corn.

Also, be aware that a high protein diet can affect the kidneys, especially if there is little to no physical activity, so again, moderation of protein intake is another matter to consider for sedentary people. A high protein diet may be appropriate for athletes because of their rigorous activity levels, but not for anyone else who doesn't engage in the same level of exercise.

Another factor to consider in designing the right carb cycling diet program is the physical conditioning of the person. Determine which activity one is engaged mostly in – mental or physical activity. Each has different nutritional requirements.

Meeting the right nutritional requirements for either mental or physical conditioning is what the carb cycling dietary program is all about. It balances the protein requirement of protein with the right amount of carbohydrates for optimum nutrition.

The Dietary Cycles

The generally accepted cycles to follow in the carb cycling dietary program are any combination of a low carb day, a moderate carb day, a high carb day and a no carb day. Although there is no fixed schedule to follow, it is recommended that in designing the best diet plan based on carb cycling, the person has to know their daily caloric requirements.

Determine which days you are the most physically active. On these days it's best to consume a high amount of carbs to provide enough energy. This can be followed by a moderate or a low carb day, in order to expend excess energy or calories that were not spent. On a lazy Sunday, a no carb or low carb diet may be the right choice. The reason is there is no need for additional energy; the stored energy in the body will be sufficient to last for such an uneventful day. Then, it may be followed by one or more moderate carb days to regulate another round of slowly building up and storing energy. These are but two examples of combining each cycle in a given week. There are more ways to combine different carb cycling days.

Any number of cycle combinations can be devised in a week such as three low carb days, two high carb days and two moderate carb days, for a very relaxed method of maintaining weight. Or if the person needs to lose weight really fast, then just having one very high carb day in seven days is good enough to do the trick. Then, after achieving the desired weight loss, going back to a more relaxed carb cycling combination would be suitable for maintaining that desired weight.

The schedule that suits you really depends on your lifestyle. If you exercise rigorously every day, then more high or moderate carb days may be required. If you're sedentary and overweight, you can have lower or no carb days. It all comes down to you and your needs.

YOUR HUNGER HORMONES

There is a hidden secret to carb cycling that people breeze over when discussing how it all works. I think understanding how to manage and manipulate your hunger hormones is vital to your weight loss, whether you are carb cycling or not.

One of America's biggest health problems is obesity, which affects more than one-third of the country's population. Because of this, scientists have taken steps to find the cause of obesity and ultimately find an ideal solution to curb appetite and prevent excessive weight gain. In 1994, Rockefeller University students found out that a hormone called leptin helps control appetite, and that weight loss can be controlled by manipulating this hormone.

Leptin, which is derived from the Greek word "leptos," essentially lives up to the name. It means "thin," and interestingly, it is a hormone manufactured by the body's fat cells. One of leptin's jobs is to tell the brain that there is enough energy stored in the body and to stop eating food.

However, most people nowadays overeat until they have reached the highest level of leptin that they can tolerate. Some people eventually get to the point when their bodies begin refusing the "you are full" signal they get from the hormone. Because of bad eating habits, the signaling capability of the hormone becomes impaired. When leptin levels become impaired, it eventually fails to stop telling the body that it has enough energy, and you experience the need to binge uncontrollably.

Overweight people tend to have impaired leptin levels, and their bodies do not recognize that they are taking in more food then they need to meet their energy needs. This is called leptin resistance and could be a big factor in obesity. If your body doesn't know when you are full, how could it not be a factor?

Leptin Resistance

What causes leptin resistance in the first place? One major reason is that we have switched our diets from that of whole food to one of highly processed goods. These processed foods are high in fructose and sugar. Certain studies prove that having high levels of triglycerides, which fructose creates, prevents leptin from efficiently sending signals to the brain. If your brain ignores the leptin signal, you feel like you haven't got enough food and just keep eating.

Leptin resistance not only causes binging but another problem, which is the creation of reverse T3. This prevents the thyroid hormone from properly stimulating your metabolism. For people who are battling with weight issues, leptin resistance offers a double whammy.

Our diets are most likely the biggest factor in developing leptin resistance. Leptin resistance develops silently, with most people being oblivious as to what is happening inside their bodies. Most people ended up overweight and confused as to why they can't seem to lose weight or curb their appetite.

You may have or be developing leptin resistance if you experience the following:

1. Uncontrollable craving for food

2. Obsession with food

3. Abnormal metabolism

4. Overeating

You should get everything back on track by following a carb cycling diet, and you may want to consult your physician if you suspect your leptin levels may be the culprit of your weight gain.

I hope you understand now how we can manipulate leptin to our advantage by keeping it stimulated through the days of our carb cycle. If you are struggling with weight loss, it could be because you have too many high carbs, low carb, or no carb days in a row. You should try to never have more than two of any one day (high, low or no) in a row. This prevents leptin levels from getting too low or too high.

Ghrelin or gremlin

When it comes to hunger, there's another hormone that you should pay attention to. This hormone is called ghrelin and is the chemical that is mostly produced to stimulate hunger, signaling the body to find food.

If you are low on leptin, then ghrelin happily takes over and tells you to eat, eat and eat. Ghrelin levels dramatically increase before meals and drop about three hours after eating. So for those who want to reduce weight, you would want more leptin and less ghrelin, as they function in inverse proportion most of the time. You can't get rid of ghrelin, but you can reduce it through carb cycling.

Having an elevated level of ghrelin in the body tends to cause a person to make the worst decisions when it comes to food. Studies show that increased ghrelin in the body makes people opt to eat foods rich in sugar and fats. That burger and fries will seem a lot more appealing then salmon and salad when ghrelin is controlling you.

I know from personal experience with carb cycling that once my leptin levels stabilized, I struggled to eat enough to keep losing weight. It may seem like a strange problem to have, but you need to keep eating in order not to become too calorie deficient. I also didn't need to fight off cravings like I thought I would. I was always a big believer that you would crave processed foods forever, but once you control your ghrelin, those cravings happen few and far between.

Getting leptin & ghrelin to play nice

Now that you understand how both leptin and ghrelin operate, let's look at some ways we can balance the two to make sure we stay in the sweet spot of fat burning. You will recognize most of these as traits following carb cycling offers.

1. Consume more protein daily. Protein effectively reduces hunger and also prolongs the length of time you can go without food. Some studies also suggest that increased amounts of protein in your diet help improve leptin sensitivity.

2. Indulge in foods rich in fiber. High amounts of fiber in the daily diet help in promoting weight loss. At the same time, having natural fiber in every meal helps in lowering one's ghrelin levels. In fact, a study showed that eating bread with fermentable fiber lowers ghrelin levels almost 25% compared to eating normal bread.

3. Get the right amount of sleep. I would have never guessed at how much of an impact sleeping would have on weight loss, but its importance cannot be ignored. Getting enough sleep actually lowers ghrelin levels and elevates leptin levels. Research has shown that people who get 7 hours of sleep or more a night have less body fat than those that don't. This could be from a number of factors, but the hormone disturbance from lack of sleep can be traced right back to your weight gain.

4. You won't escape the benefits of healthy fats. If you do not like eating fish, you may want to rethink that or try the fish oil supplements we discussed earlier. Omega 3's found in fish oil may help combat leptin resistance. You can also incorporate walnuts and other similar nuts into your diet since they are also rich in Omega 3 fatty acids.

5. Ensure your weekly calorie intake is not too low. Your cravings and ghrelin will shoot through the roof if you are not getting the right amount of calories needed for your daily tasks and workouts. Our goal with carb cycling is to end up in a calorie deficit at the end of each cycle but not to the point that we are starving our bodies.

6. Avoid skipping meals. The more meals you skip, the fewer calories you take in, which we said could spike your ghrelin. Your body's leptin levels also shift to be timed with the meals that you consistently eat. Skipping a meal would make your leptin delay doing its job. While that happens, the amount of ghrelin produced in your body is greatly increased every 20 to 30 minutes. If you

know you are not going to be able to eat a snack or meal at your regular time, a protein shake or green smoothie may save the day.

7. Have a healthier gut. There is growing evidence being produced that obesity may be linked to an imbalance in the healthy bacteria in our stomach. They are years away from producing a bacteria pill for weight loss, but in the meantime, we can do our part. You may want to consider adding fermented foods into your meals, like sauerkraut or kimchi, to get a dose of healthy bacteria. You can also choose to supplement with a probiotic if you feel it is needed.

8. Reduce stress. This may seem like a no-brainer, but most people have come to believe that being stressed is normal. It isn't, and that stress could be adding to the pounds as you read this. Chances have you have stressed already about your weight, which is why you are reading a weight loss book. Stress causes hormone imbalances in the body and leads to overeating. How often do you deal with stress by reaching for a tossed salad instead of Combo #1? Not too often for most people.

Like everything in life, the best results stem from finding a balance. We need leptin and ghrelin in our diets and life, obviously, but they need to work in harmony. We can do our part by choosing carb cycling as our method of dieting and taking note of the above tips. Never discount the importance of the small things when it comes to weight loss.

I hope by understanding your hunger hormones better, you can use them to your advantage in your weight loss. It only takes small changes in your diet to make big changes in the numbers on the scale.

What About Cardio?

Cardio is a very hot topic in the fitness community today. You hear about professional bodybuilders using it to lean down for competitions, but then you hear someone else bashing it for being too slow and boring.

So, who's right in all of this? Hopefully, I can set you on the right path and give you a true understanding of what cardio is all about.

Is Cardio Even Necessary to Lose Weight?

The answer to the above question is definitely not! I can completely understand why many people think that they must do hours upon hours of cardio if they want to shed a few pounds. You hear all of the time about how fitness models and bodybuilders use cardio as a way to get absolutely shredded, so it's easy to believe it's required. However, cardio is not required at all to lose weight and get down to a low level of body fat.

What is required to lose weight and shred fat is eating fewer calories than your total daily energy expenditure. It doesn't matter if you use exercise (i.e., cardio in this case) and/or diet to achieve that, both will get the job done. With that being said, it's much easier to control your total number of calories through your diet as opposed to exercising more. Think about it for a second.

What's easier- eating a slice of pizza and then doing 30 minutes of cardio to burn it off or not eating the slice of pizza in the first place? It's obvious; you shouldn't eat the pizza in the first place. Sure, you could try to burn off the extra calories every now and then, but it won't last for long. You're fighting an uphill battle because 30 minutes of your time isn't worth whatever it is that you want to eat so badly.

That's why you hear people say that you can't out exercise a bad diet. It's true, so focus more on your diet and the number of calories that you're eating instead of doing more cardio. Also, don't fret if you think this means that you'll have to give up your favorite foods to lose weight because it doesn't. You'll still get to enjoy your favorite foods *without* having to worry about weight gain or doing some extra cardio to make up for it.

How You Should Think About Cardio

From now on, I want you to think about cardio as a tool that can help you burn some extra calories instead of thinking of cardio as

64

a requirement to do with carb cycling to lose weight. Cardio is one way to help get you below your total daily energy expenditure (TDEE), and you can use it when you feel that it's needed to get the job done.

As a single tool usually won't be enough to get the job done, cardio alone usually won't be enough to get you burning more calories than your TDEE. The main focus still needs to be on the carb cycling nutrition plan I outlined earlier. With this type of mindset, you'll only have to do cardio when you feel that it's necessary. It's important to note that moderate to high-intensity cardio *isn't required* at all for carb cycling to work.

I believe that honing in on nutrition is the right way to go when trying to lose weight. This is because the diet is the easiest and fastest way to control the total number of calories you're eating. However, once you have your diet in check if you feel like adding in some extra exercise, then, by all means, do so. Cardio can be a good way to speed up the fat loss process or at the very least give you some more leeway in your diet.

The Best Cardio Workout

With so many cardio workouts in existence today, which one is the best? Is it slow, steady state cardio? How about sprinting? Or maybe any type of cardio done on an empty stomach is the best?

The kind of cardio that you do doesn't matter much. This is because if the cardio workout doesn't put your total caloric intake below your TDEE (I know I keep bringing this up so it must be important, right?), then you won't be losing any weight.

So, I would first and foremost recommend doing any type of cardio you enjoy, whether that's walking, sprinting, jogging, swimming, kickboxing, etc. However, I will say the cardio workout I'll be providing you with here is the best way to go. It's a combination of high-intensity interval training (HIIT) and slows steady state cardio. Research has shown higher intensity cardio results in fatter loss over time than lower intensity cardio.

HIIT really is efficient—you're burning more calories in less time. HIIT's even cooler though when combined with slow, steady state cardio. The reason why is because the HIIT will release free fatty acids into the bloodstream, and then the slow, steady state cardio will burn off those free fatty acids.

Most people will do HIIT but won't follow it up with slow, steady state cardio. This is a shame because all of those free fatty acids released into the bloodstream will get reabsorbed.

Here's how to do a combo cardio workout

Note: This cardio workout can be done on any type of cardio machine (treadmill, elliptical, etc.), outside, on a track or wherever else you want. No matter where you are, the workout will be the same.

Combo Cardio Workout

#1: 10-15 minutes of HIIT on the treadmill (or cardio machine of choice)

-Sprint for 30 seconds

-Walk for 1 minute (alternate between sprinting and walking for the full 10-15 min)

#2: Immediately followed by 10-15 minutes of steady state cardio

-Walk on the treadmill at 3.5 mph

Now the cool thing about HIIT is that you can adjust it to your current fitness level. For example, if you can't sprint for 30 seconds, do a fast jog for 20 seconds (7.5 mph on a treadmill as an example) and then walk for 1 minute and 10 seconds.

You could even do 45 seconds of sprinting and 45 seconds of walking if you're in better shape. You can customize it to your needs, but you have the do the HIIT first followed by the slow, steady state cardio.

I recommend that you do this 20-30-minute workout 2 times per week. I wouldn't advise that you do it any more than 2 times per week because that's too much and it's not necessary beyond that point.

Final Cardio Considerations

Here's the deal:

You might not feel like doing HIIT sometimes. What do you do then? Luckily, you don't have to skip cardio altogether—there's an easier way, and it's called walking. I recommend walking as much as you possibly can.

Walking is great because it can help to reduce stress and speed up recovery from a hard workout. Walking also helps with lymphatic system recovery, and there's research showing how walking more (or moving more in general for that matter) can reduce your risk for developing heart disease.

Best of all, walking is an easy way to burn more calories. I used to think that walking was only for people who weren't in that good of shape, but boy was I wrong about that! Walking should be done by everyone, fit, or unfit. The simple fact is that walking provides benefits that the higher intensity cardio can't.

I recommend going for walks around town or at the local park. Go outside and get some fresh air. Walking for 30 minutes, 3 days a week would be enough to start providing you with some amazing benefits. You can still do the combination cardio workout twice per week in addition to the walking if you want to.

Carb Cycling

and Weight Loss

As a new diet, this diet is somewhat developed from the factors that undergird manipulating carbs. As such, there are still not many substantiated and controlled studies that directly investigate a carb cycling routine. In basic terms, carb cycling is a mechanism through which we try to match our body's requirement for glucose or calories.

Theoretically, this method will certainly maximize the overall benefits that carbs offer our bodies. As explained in the earlier part of this text, the benefits that carbs give our bodies is immense. While the factors that support cycling carbs certainly support its implementation, it should be viewed with some caution due to a lack of direct research about its complete effect on our health. However, this is mainly pertinent for individuals that have a history of medical concerns, especially those that have had concerns and issues related to diets that they have implemented.

Here are some important things that you should keep in mind before fully implementing the carb-cycling diet into your routine for any period of time:

Days of High-Carb Consumption Are to Be Implemented on Intense Training Days:

Perhaps the most important thing that you should be aware of as it pertains to this to carb cycling is that you should put your highest carb consumption on days where you plan on having your most intense workout sessions. So, for instance, this means that you should be eating the most carbs on heavy workout days, or on days that involve a full body workout. This is because our bodies require carbohydrates at our most intense levels on these specific times of the week. Moreover, consuming these prior to exercising will give your body enough fuel so that you have enough energy to push your way through the most challenging aspects of the workout. Thereafter, having carbs right after the workout will help replenish and nourish your body so that you recover fast and that your body has enough energy to have another intense workout the next day or later in the week. Specifically, this is also great for building more muscle as it will allow you to lift more weight for longer periods of time.

Because you want your carb consumption to be put to the best use possible in a manner that allows you to maximize results, along with preventing them from being converted into body fat, you have to ensure that you are timing them correctly throughout the course of the week. Planning your carb cycling, in this way, is an integral part of making sure that this method works best for you. Coupled with already having knowledge about how your body works and strategies work best for training and exercising your body, planning your intake of carbs in a strategic manner is key to getting the absolute most out of your body while training or, more generally, in your everyday life.

You May Gain Water Weight

You should also be aware of, and prepare for, possibly gaining a little bit of weight at times of implementing the high-carb day. With every carb that is consumed, your body will then hold on to 4g of water. So, when consuming 250- 350g of carbs on days high-carb intake, this will tend to add up extremely quickly.

For people whose body composition is already leaner, they will experience this effect mostly due to water weight simply being more noticeable on their leaner body. Not to worry, this is a completely a common process. And, thankfully, this excess water weight does not signal that your body is gaining fat. This kind of weight gain will certainly recede within a few days on the normal low-carb intake regimen.

Now, it is important to be aware of whether you are someone who struggles with weight gain from a psychological perspective. If this is you, then perhaps cycling carbs is dangerous for you and you should reconsider. Indeed, temporary water weight gain tends to common accompany this dietary routine. Moreover, be prepared for this to take place prior to undertaking the diet possibly.

Select Carbs That Are Highest in Complex Carbohydrates or Glucose

As it pertains to selecting which food to consume when undertaking a carb cycling regimen for losing fat, you need to consider glucose. This includes either source of simple glucose (which should be consumed somewhere near the workout period where they will incidentally be absorbed much faster) or complex carbs that will be broken into glucose by your body naturally.

What should be avoided in this instance is fructose (as in high-fructose corn syrup to be specific), because this form of carb will interact differently with your body and will not have any of the positive benefits that accompany glucose.

If, for example, you consume a lot of fructose during periods of high-carb consumption, there is a high likelihood that it will be turned into fat because it will not be stored within your muscles as quickly.

Lower Your Fat Consumption on During High-Carb

One of the integral consideration to bear in mind as you integrate a carb cycling regimen is that you need to decrease your fat intake on high-carb days. However, by lowering the overall fat intake, you will be allowing greater space for these carbs without consuming too many total calories.

In an ideal plan, you should try to stay within a 350-600 overall calorie limit on your days of low-carb intake in order to prevent the consumption of excess calories from being in a stalemate with your fat loss for that particular week.

Sustain Your Weekly Target Calorie Level for Losing Fat

As an appendage of the point above is that the overall week intake of calories should remain at a level that is needed for losing fat.

For instance, when keeping your weight at 2300 calories per day, which is just slightly more than 15,400 per week, you will need to trigger an overall calorie deficit of 3500 calories per week or consume 11,900 total calories/week in order to shed one pound per week.

Standard diets require you to maintain a similar calorie level on every day of the week, this- requires you to consume 1700 calories/day. Now, consider whether you wanted to have 3 high-carb days to maximize the benefits and get the most results, you should set the calorie intake at 2400— just make sure that your weekly protein consumption remains consistent all week. As a result, because those 3 days equal nearly 7200 total calories, you will have 4700 calories that are remaining for the remaining 4 days, which is nearly 1100 calories for each.

You might be able to tell that these low carb days are very low in calories; however, following high-carb days, many people will find this to be rather easy and not too much of a struggle. If, for instance, you would rather not bring you low-carb days too low on the total amount of calorie that you consume, all you really have to do is bring the overall intake of calories on high-carb days lower. As a result, you will get more calories for low-carb days as well. This is significant because it demonstrates that you can certainly tinker and adjust your carb cycling in a manner that works best for you. This diet regimen is not overly stringent and strenuous insofar as it limits your capacity to play around with the math. Rather, you are able to adjust the calorie and carb levels to such a degree that you reap the most benefits without having to sacrifice comfort or put too much of a strain on your body and the way that you feel.

You can probably tell that the idea of carb cycling is really about balance. Finding ways to balance your intake of carbs and calories will enhance your overall enjoyment and the benefits that you enjoy from the diet. Just be sure that your weekly intake of carbs and calories is exactly where it needs to be and that you alter and adjust accordingly. After you establish your preferences, make sure that you start to distribute all of your calories thereafter.

Getting Past the Fat-Burning Plateau

One of the telltale signs of reaching a fat-burning plateau is when you see no progress in your body no matter how hard you grind at the gym. If not addressed properly, you can go on for weeks exercising at the gym and will still get no results.

Reaching a wall during a diet or workout is very common, and almost all people who diet and work out at the gym experience this. As a person approaches his ideal weight, his body will be more resistant to change; thus, the arrival of the fat-burning plateau. The concept is just simple, really. Since the body becomes leaner, there will be lesser excess fats to burn. This will cause your weight loss progress to slow down and eventually stops when your body has fully adjusted to your workout and diet routine.

When going on a low-carb diet, you will reduce the intake of carbohydrates for a certain period of time, which will then result in losing water weight and a substantial amount of body fats.

What many don't know is that the longer the body is deprived of carbohydrates, the slower their metabolism becomes until they reach a wall. Once carbohydrates are reintroduced, the body then goes on the rebound, which will make it more difficult to lose weight and body fats again.

With carb cycling, a dieter will never have to worry about reaching a fat-burning plateau. Since carb cycling has carbohydrate refill days, the body's carb supply will never be low enough to slow metabolism. Also, during low-carb days, the body enters a state of catabolic fat burning, which ensures that the person loses unwanted body fats throughout the duration of the diet. In short, the high-carb days serves as a metabolism booster in order for the body to burn more fats during low-carb days.

The changing level of nutrients in carb cycling keeps the body "guessing" and prevents it from going into a metabolic downshift which commonly happens to linear type of diets. Another good strategy to get past the plateau is by injecting a week of high-carb diet every three weeks of carb cycling. Changing your eating pattern will not only trick your metabolism but will also prepare your body to absorb and use these nutrients to increase your body build. Implementing periodical changes in your diet will go a long way in ensuring that you don't hit a wall during your program.

Carb Cycling

and Health Concerns

If you want to try carb cycling, then there are certain things that you need to keep in mind.

Never Ignore your Thyroid

The thyroid is an essential hormone for fat loss. However, on a low carb diet, the production of the thyroid will slow down in the body. When the production of thyroid slows down, it can cause problems with a woman's metabolic system. Women are more sensitive to the behavior of the thyroid than men. An imbalance in the thyroid hormone can lead to hypothyroidism. So, how can you avoid it? It is quite simple. You need to make sure that your body gets at least 50 grams of carbs on any given day. It is quite easy to include 50 grams of carbs in your daily meal. Never scrimp on carbs, if you don't want to harm your thyroid secretion in the body. Did you know that something as simple as one large sweet potato contains 50 grams of carbs?

Menstrual Cycle

Two hormones that influence carbohydrate metabolism in women are estrogen and progesterone. Estrogen can increase insulin sensitivity, and progesterone tends to decrease insulin sensitivity in the body. During the first two weeks of the cycle or the follicular phase, the body can process carbs more efficiently than during the last two weeks of the cycle. The last two weeks of the cycle are the ones after ovulation, and during this period, when the body starts to process carbs, most of it is stored in the form of fat in the body. Therefore, be mindful of your menstrual cycle while you decide the low and the high carb days. If you place most of your high carb days during the last two weeks of your monthly cycle, your body will not burn carbs efficiently, and it will lead to fat gain in the body.

Starvation Mode

When you opt for carb cycling, you need to ensure that your diet lets you consume a sufficient amount of calories. Most women tend to think that a low-calorie diet is more effective than other forms of diet. If you don't consume sufficient calories and skimp on carbs while you exercise, then it will harm your body's ability to regulate the reproductive hormones in your body. If you skimp on calories as well as carbs, then your body can misinterpret this as external stress. While under stress, the body shuts down the reproductive system. It doesn't matter if this so-called "stress" is voluntary. Your body cannot differentiate between a self-imposed calorie deficit and one caused due to starvation. It will affect your reproductive health if you aren't mindful of all that you eat.

A woman's body is relatively more sensitive to the signals of starvation than that of a man. So, whenever your body notices a decrease in your food intake, it tends to misinterpret the same as starvation and in turn, increases the production of leptin and ghrelin. Leptin and ghrelin are the two hormones that trigger hunger. When there is an increase in the secretion of these chemical compounds, you will experience extreme hunger. Technically, your body doesn't need any extra food, but it is merely your hormones that tell you otherwise. Whenever a woman's body feels that it is headed towards a famine (intentional or not), it increases the secretion of the hunger hormones. The hunger hormones, as is obvious from the name, signal your body to increase the intake of food. Also, if there isn't enough food to survive, then your body will start to shut its reproductive system. A woman's body will not want to procreate when it feels like there isn't sufficient sustenance to nourish itself. In fact, it is the body's natural defense against a potential pregnancy during famines. Your body will protect itself from pregnancy, regardless of whether you want to conceive or not.

Your body cannot differentiate between a self-imposed fast and a famine. Therefore, the body cannot differentiate between starvation and calorie reduction. That is why the default protective mechanism kicks in.

Success Tips

Human bodies are quite efficient. You can adapt your body to different training programs within no time. If there is no change in physical stimuli, then your body tends to stay the same. However, if you eat the same foods all the time, it will hit a plateau in your progress. The best manner in which you can encourage your body to change is to alter your diet periodically. If you want your body to burn fats to provide energy or create a meal plan that better suits your energy needs, then carb cycling is the simple answer. Carb cycling is simple, and all that you need to do is alter your carb intake daily. In this section, you will learn about a couple of tips that will help you along the way.

Don't Skip Meals

Do you tend to skip meals? Regardless of how busy you might be, you always have the time for a quick meal. Don't skip any meals. Your body needs glucose to function, and glucose is obtained by breaking down the carbs that you consume. So, when you skip a meal, you deny your body the fuel that it needs to function, and this leads to imbalances in your blood sugar levels. When your blood sugar is low, you will feel dizzy and lightheaded. It also affects your mood. When your brain doesn't get sufficient glucose, it cannot function optimally. It can lead to mood swings, and you will be irritable. You can easily remedy this; you just need to make it a point to eat. Skipping meals increases your risk of diabetes. It happens because of the delay in your body's response to processing insulin when you don't have timely meals. All this is bound to harm your metabolism. When you skip meals, your body automatically shifts into starvation mode and starts slowing down its metabolism. If you are trying to lose weight by skipping meals, you are merely sabotaging your weight loss program. It leads to acid reflux and can result in ulcers and severe abdominal pain.

Don't Overeat

You need to have well-balanced meals. You must not skip your meals, but this doesn't mean that you need to overeat either. Eat only when you are hungry and stop yourself from eating unnecessarily. Here are a couple of simple things that you can do to avoid overeating.

Learn to eat slowly. It certainly isn't a new concept, but not many follow it. We are all in a hurry these days. Take a moment and slow down. Take a sip of water between bites and chew your food thoroughly before swallowing it. Don't just gulp down your food; learn to chew it slowly. Start paying attention to what you are eating. Savor the food you are eating and don't just stuff yourself with food. Think about the different textures and flavors. Savor every bite you eat and make it a pleasurable experience. Make your first bites count and satisfy your taste buds. Make use of a smaller plate; this will enable you to control the portions you eat visually thinking you have already eaten enough as opposed to using a larger plate. Stay away from foods that are rich in calories but do nothing to satisfy your appetite. Choose foods that will fill you up; foods that are satisfying. Foods rich in protein and fiber will fill your tummy. Instead of having a bar of chocolate or a pint of ice cream, have a portion of meat with grilled vegetables. This will satiate your hunger. Food that is rich in calories makes you feel full for a while, but you will be hungry within an hour. This results in overeating. By being mindful of what you are eating, you can stop yourself from overeating. While eating, make it a point to stay away from all electronic gadgets. This means no television or mobile gadgets. The next time you are bored, don't reach out for the box of cookies or the bag of chips. Think before indulging in mindless eating; the results will be worth it!

Drink Plenty of Water

Water is good for your body, and drinking plenty of water will make your skin clearer and will flush out all of the toxins from your body. Make it a habit to have at least 8 glasses of water daily. If you want to, you can add some flavorings or electrolytes to your water to spruce it up. Slices of lemon, different berries, a handful of mint leaves, or slices of cucumber can be added to water for making detox water. By following these five simple tips, you can trick yourself into drinking water.

Drinking water needs to be convenient. Carry a water bottle or a sipper with yourself wherever you go. If a water bottle is handy, it is more likely that you will drink water without a reminder. Instead of sugary sodas and sweetened beverages, you can have unsweetened water-based drinks. Instead of a Frappuccino, have a cup of Americano. Make it a point to drink a glass of water before and after your meals. Set a goal and measure the amount of water you are drinking daily. If you keep track of your water intake, you will be motivated to drink more. Don't forget to drink water even when you go out drinking with your friends. Don't let your body get dehydrated.

Whole Grains are Good for You

At least half of the grains you consume must be whole-grains. Examples of whole grains are barley, brown rice, oatmeal, popcorn, bulgur, buckwheat, and millet. Replace the regular grains you consume with whole grains and wholegrain products. Instead of regular pasta, buy wholegrain pasta. It tastes the same and is much better for your health. Check the labels before you buy something to make sure that you are buying wholegrain produce. These grains help in improving your heart's health, can reduce the risk of certain cancers, quite helpful in managing diabetes, and helps in managing your weight as well.

Be Mindful of What You Eat

Always make sure that you increase the intake of leafy vegetables on low-carb days. Leafy greens are rich in fiber, and it will make you feel fuller for a longer period of time. Even if your calorie intake is low, you will not feel hungry if you fill yourself up with a generous serving of leafy greens. On the low-carb days, your main source of energy will be from whole-foods. Whole foods include foods that are naturally full of healthy fats like avocados, eggs, coconut oil, fish caught in the wild, nuts, and grass-fed butter.

You need to measure your intake of fats and carbs. If you want to stick to carb cycling, then it is important that you stay within the ideal levels of proper carb and fat intake. It will not do your body any good if you overestimate your carb intake and underestimate the intake of protein.

If you want to reduce your carb intake on moderate-carb and low-carb days, then you need to increase your intake of fats. You must never eliminate one macronutrient without substituting it with another source. Your body needs either fats or carbs to generate energy. If you deplete your body of both the sources of energy, it will shift to starvation mode. Be mindful of the macros you feed your body on the days you exercise.

Keep these simple tips in mind when you follow carb cycling. It will certainly make your diet much more effective.

Frequently Asked Questions

Can I Treat My High-Carb Days Like a Cheat Day?

No, you can't. There's a difference between a high-carb day and a cheat day. A cheat day brings with it the mentality that you can eat whatever you want whenever you want. This can make things get out of hand at times, causing you to overeat. A high-carb day, on the other hand, is a strategic part of the carb cycling process. You're still limited to eating a moderate amount of fat, and you'll want the majority of your carbs to come from quality food sources.

What if I'm not losing or gaining weight eating 13 calories per pound of bodyweight?

If you've been struggling to lose weight, eating 13 calories per pound of body weight, then I recommend using a different method to set your calories. Before I get into that though, you must first make sure you were actually eating 13 calories per pound of bodyweight minus 500 calories to lose 1 pound per week. It's easy to overestimate the number of calories you're eating, and this could be the reason why you do not see results.

Once you've made sure you've accurately been tracking your calories, you can take your goal bodyweight, multiply it by 11 and then eat that many calories (don't subtract anything from the final calculated number).

Yes, I understand that your goal bodyweight will be a random number that you think you'll look good at, so take your best guess. Start on the higher side and work your way down from there if you still aren't losing weight.

Here's an example of a 250-pound male.

Current Weight 250

Goal Bodyweight 200

200 x 11= 2,200 daily calories

Let's say once this person reaches his goal of 200 pounds, he's still not satisfied with how he looks. From there, he can simply set a new goal bodyweight (i.e., 190 pounds, for example) and go from there.

On the other hand, let's say you're struggling to add muscle eating 13 calories per pound of bodyweight plus 250 calories. Again, make sure you're accurately tracking the amount of calories you're eating. You could be miscounting your calories, and that would account for why you're not gaining any weight. Once you've made sure you're tracking things accurately, you can add 100 calories to your total resting metabolic rate weekly until you start gaining weight. For example:

A 180-pound male looking to gain weight would multiply his bodyweight by 13 to determine his maintenance calories.

180 x 13= 2,340

This person would then add 250 calories to 2,340 and get a total of 2,590 calories per day. If he eats 2,590 calories on a daily basis, he should start to gain 0.5 pounds per week. However, if he doesn't, he can simply add 100 calories to his original 2,590 calories on a weekly basis until he does.

For example, in week 1, he would eat 2,690 calories. If he didn't gain any weight by the end of the week, he would eat 2,790 calories for the following week, and so on and so forth until he starts gaining weight.

What if I hit a plateau and I stop losing weight at my regular pace?

Let's say you've been losing weight just fine, but then all of a sudden you hit a wall and stop losing weight. In this case, take your new current bodyweight (which should be a lower number from when you first started) and multiply that by 13.

Take that number and subtract 250 from it. This will be your new daily caloric intake for you to lose weight.

This will have you losing weight at a rate of approximately 0.5 pounds per week. You may have previously been losing weight at a rate of 1 pound per week, but now you'll lose at a rate of 0.5 pounds per week.

This is because I don't want you to reduce your calories all of a sudden drastically and because if you've hit a plateau, you're likely very close to hitting your goal weight anyway.

How many meals should I eat per day?

You can eat as many meals as you like throughout the day. Meal frequency doesn't matter for weight loss, but the total amount of calories you eat does. So eat, however, is easiest for you and your schedule.

I, myself, prefer to eat 3 meals a day and that works great for most people. However, feel free to eat 6 times per day or even as little as once per day. As long as you're hitting your macros, you'll be fine.

What do I do once I reach my goal bodyweight?

Contrary to what you might be thinking, things aren't going to be that much different from what you've been doing to lose weight. You still need to do flexible dieting and continue eating in the same manner that you previously were. This means that you should still keep the same eating schedule and keep eating similar meals to the ones that you were eating to lose weight.

However, there's one difference between maintenance and creating a caloric deficit to lose weight. The difference is that you get to consume more calories! How many calories? Well, this is pretty easy to figure out as a matter of fact.

Step #1: Determine at what rate you were losing weight (i.e., 1 pound per week).

Step #2: Translate pounds lost per week into calories.

- 0.5 pound lost per week= 250 calories

- 1 pound lost per week= 500 calories

- 1.5 pounds lost per week= 750 calories

- 2 pounds lost per week= 1,000 calories, etc.

Step #3: Add in those additional calories to what you were previously eating to maintain your new weight.

For example, let's say someone was losing weight at a rate of 1 pound per week by eating 1,850 calories per day. Once he hits his goal weight, he needs to eat 2,350 calories (1,850+500) per day to maintain his new weight.

You'll also need to recalculate your macro percentages. Continuing with this example, this individual would need to do the following with his new caloric intake:

- 2,350 x .40= 940 daily calories from protein

- 2,350 x .35= 822.5 daily calories from carbs

- 2,350 x .25= 587.5 daily calories from fat

How much weight should I lift during the workouts?

Lift as much weight as you possibly can for the given rep range. Initially, you won't know how much weight to use, so you'll have to take your best guess. For example, let's say you're doing bench press for 8 reps. You think you can lift around 150 pounds for that many reps, but on your first set, you easily complete 10 reps.

This means the weight is too light and you need to increase it for the next set. On the next set, you lift 165 pounds and struggle to complete the 8th rep. This is what you want to happen, and it means you've found a good weight to use. Once you can complete all 3 sets for 8 reps with 165 pounds, move up to 170 the next time you bench press. If you can't complete 8 reps for all 3 sets, stick with 165 until you can. Here's an example:

Workout 1: Bench Press with 165 pounds

- Set 1: 8 reps

- Set 2: 8 reps

- Set 3: 7 reps

Because you only completed 7 reps on the last set, stick with 165 for the next workout.

Workout 2: Bench Press with 165 pounds

- Set 1: 8 reps

- Set 2: 8 reps

- Set 3: 8 reps

Because you completed all 3 sets for 8 reps, move up to 170 on your next workout with the bench press.

Note: It's better to use a weight that's too heavy and miss a rep or two than it is to use a weight that's too light and leave some reps in the tank. For example, it's better to do 170 pounds and only complete 6 reps instead of 8 as opposed to using 155 pounds and stopping at 8 reps even though you could've easily done more reps.

How Fast Should I Lose Weight?

The more weight you have to lose, the faster the rate at which you can lose the weight. For example, if you have 50+ pounds to lose, you can lose weight at a rate of 2 pounds or more per week. If you only have 5 pounds to lose, then lose weight at a rate of 0.5 pounds per week.

For most people, losing 1 pound per week is the sweet spot. You'll be creating an average caloric deficit of 500 calories daily. At this pace, you'll be losing weight fairly quickly, and you won't be miserable all of the time from a complete lack of calories.

How much water should I drink on a daily basis?

Your body is made up of about 60% water, so it's important to consume water for several reasons. Drinking water regularly:

Helps keep your joints and ligaments fluid, which can help prevent injury

- Helps control your caloric intake

- Flushes out toxins

- Improves skin quality

- Improves kidney function

- Improves your focus

Many people recommend that you should drink 1 gallon of water per day. This is a blanket answer that doesn't meet individual needs. This recommendation would have a 100-pound woman drinking the same amount of water as a 200-pound man. Absurd!

Other health experts advise drinking eight 8-ounce glasses (64 ounces total) of water a day. But again 64 ounces isn't going to be enough for most people. What should you do then? I don't keep track of my water intake—I go by how I feel and the color of my urine.

Your body's own thirst mechanism will be accurate in telling you if you need more water. If you feel thirsty, go drink some water. If not, you're probably ok. You can also use the color of your urine to judge how hydrated you are. If your urine is yellow, then you should drink more water. If it's clear, then you should be good to go. This keeps things simple, and it's one less thing you have to keep track of.

Are there any supplements that you recommend I take?

Most supplements are a complete waste of money. There's not a single supplement that's required in order for you to build muscle or burn fat. In fact, I advise for the first 6 weeks of your IIFYM diet that you don't take *any* supplements at all.

This is because I want you to see for yourself that it really is possible for you to get results without supplements. Your hard work and dedication matter way more than any pill or powder.

With that being said, there are a few supplements I recommend if you have the budget for them:

#1: Protein Powder:

You can't have a recommended list of supplements without protein powder on the list, right? Just kidding. But this has to be one of the most overhyped supplements of all time.

I think that the media does a really good job of making us believe that we must take protein powder to build muscle or take it to prevent muscle loss. I do think that protein powder can provide some benefits if *you need it.*

If you struggle to hit your macros with protein consistently, then I would consider investing in a protein powder. Protein is necessary to help build and prevent the breakdown of muscle.

Therefore, ensuring that your muscle is spared is a good thing. However, don't go out of your way and eat more calories just for the sake of consuming more protein.

#2: Fish/Krill Oil

These oils are great sources of Omega-3 fatty acids. This is a good thing because most people consume too many Omega-6 fatty acids with foods like vegetable and canola oil.

Ideally, you want to be consuming a 1 to 1 ratio of Omega-3's to Omega-6's. Fish and krill oil can help you narrow the gap between the two types of fatty acids that you're consuming.

The main benefit of consuming these oils is that they act as an anti-inflammatory in your body. When you consume Omega-6's on the other hand, they act as an inflammatory.

That's why it's important to strike a balance with both of the fatty acids. The anti-inflammatory benefit is great because it can reduce your risk of developing heart disease or high blood pressure.

Finally, reducing inflammation can aid in muscle recovery. If you're going to invest in fish or krill oil, make sure that it's a very high-grade supplement.

The way that some of the lower quality oils are processed inhibits the absorption of them, which would make them completely useless — as for investing in fish or krill oil, taking either one is fine really.

Krill oil does contain the antioxidant astaxanthin, which helps with joint health, boosts cognitive function, and helps promote a healthy cholesterol balance, while fish oil does not. However, I have noticed that krill oil can be harder to find, and it's typically more expensive, so don't sweat not buying it.

#3: Digestive Enzymes

This is my favorite supplement of all time, and it's probably one of the most underrated supplements as well. If your body can't absorb the vitamins and nutrients that you're consuming, then what's the point?

The sad fact of the matter is that when our foods get cooked, many of the enzymes get destroyed. Digestive enzymes will not only help to replenish those enzymes missed from cooked foods, but it will also help your body to better break down and utilize the nutrients that you're eating.

Also, if you ever suffer regularly from bloating, heartburn or have bad skin, give digestive enzymes a try and see if you notice a difference. Of course, it's important to note that these enzymes need to be high quality if you want them to be of any use.

Simply going to the local grocery store and purchasing a $10 bottle of enzymes isn't going to cut it. You must buy a high-quality enzyme if you want to get any use out of it. Personally, I recommend using the Bio Trust.

How Do I Motivate Myself to Go to the Gym?

Finding the motivation to go to the gym or eat right can be hard. No matter who you are, there will be times when you don't feel like working out. Having that feeling is ok, but you can't let it control you. There will be times when you'll have to do it anyway even when you don't feel like it.

That's what will ultimately separate a long-term successful fitness journey from failing at it. I do have some tips to help you out along the way:

Tip #1: Focus on Gradual Improvements

Many people make fitness an all-or-nothing game. They tell themselves that they'll work out 5 days a week and eat clean 100% of the time for the rest of their lives. Let's say you workout only 4 days one week. Are you a failure?

Of course not! You still worked out 4 days, but in your mind, you are because you failed to reach 5 workouts. You make it hard to celebrate any small successes that you do have because the standards are too high.

Instead, focus on making smaller, more gradual improvements and celebrate any successes you have along the way. For example, start off with a goal to only workout 2 days per week if it's been years since you've last worked out. Once you achieve that goal, you'll feel good about yourself then you can move up to working out 3 days per week and so on.

Tip #2: Action Leads to Motivation

People think they have to get the inspiration or motivation from somewhere in order to take action necessary to work out. The reverse of that is actually true. You need to start by taking action no matter how small. And once you get started, you'll likely want to continue on with what you're doing.

When I think about everything I have to do to workout such as put my gym clothes on, drive to the gym, workout with a bunch of grueling exercises, drive back and shower, I start to make up silly excuses as to why I should skip this time. Instead, I'll tell myself to do just one exercise when I get to the gym and not pressure myself to do anything more. After I finish that first exercise, it's always easier for me to finish the rest of the workout.

You just have to get started. Try this out for any healthy habit you want to start. For example, if you want to start flossing your teeth, tell yourself you'll only floss one tooth and don't pressure yourself to do anything more than that!

Tip #3: Put Your Own Money on the Line

Money is a very powerful motivator. And you can use your own money to motivate yourself to start working out more. Here's what you're going to do—give someone a good amount of money. Not $20, but something that would actually hurt you—$100, $200, $500, or whatever you can't afford to lose.

Then tell your friend that if you don't go to the gym 3 days this week, for example, they get to keep the money. When you give up the money in the first place, you'll fight to get it back. This is much different than telling yourself you'll give the money to someone after you miss your workouts.

It's too easy to make an excuse and not give away the money. Give the money up in the first place and make sure your friend actually holds you accountable to it. This is by far the best way to get the motivation to workout. There's a real cost involved if you don't comply. You'll either get ripped or go broke trying.

Foods to Eat, Foods to Avoid

Now that you have been acquainted with scaling your current diet into a carb cycling diet, it's time to learn what food to eat and what to avoid. This is because there are different kinds of carbohydrates, proteins, and fats that you can get from the food you eat. A carb-cycling diet requires you to measure the exact amounts of these nutrients that you take. However, it's not just about the quantity. You also need to mind the quality.

Carbohydrates

Let's start with carbs. Carbohydrates are the body's primary source of energy. Whatever diet, they are an integral part of keeping your body healthy. That's why they should always be a part of your diet.

There are simple and complex carbs. This is determined by their chemical composition and how the body processes them. In general, complex carbohydrates are better than simple ones. This is because complex carbs take longer for your body to break down, so they provide even energy. But this isn't ideal in the context of carb-cycling. Simple carbs are easier to digest, so it would be used fast as you work out. But in many cases, they just don't provide real value for your body. So, choosing the right carbohydrates for carb-cycling isn't just a matter of choosing between simple and complex carbs. There are other factors that come in as to what makes certain carbs ideal while others should be avoided.

Fruits and vegetables contain simple carbohydrates – simple sugars. What makes them different is that they are high in fiber. Fiber alters the way how the human body breaks down the carbs they contain. That makes them good sources of carbohydrates.

There are more scientific details about the factors that make certain carbohydrates good or bad. But we won't go through them all at length. For this book's purposes, a list of the foods to eat and foods to avoid would be enough. There will be brief explanations following some of the items.

Good Carbs

Here are good carb sources for a carb cycling diet.

- Milk – It has lactose, a good simple carb. Just be sure that you go for low-fat or zero-fat milk, so you don't throw off the fat consumption part of your diet.

- White or Sweet Potato – Potatoes can satiate you faster, meaning you feel full faster, especially when boiled. The carbs are simple, and they contain fiber.

- Fruits – The reasons have been touched already. Carbs are especially good for berries.

- Quinoa – This is really nice for the high carb days. You'll need starchy carbs like what quinoa has during these days in the cycle.

- Oatmeal

- Whole Grain Bread

- Tortillas

- Whole Wheat Pasta

- Brown Rice

Bad Carbs

Many foods contain junk carbs. Here are some things that you have to avoid when under a carb cycling diet.

- Pastries (such as doughnuts)

- Instant oatmeal (as they tend to contain a lot of sugar)

- Pizza

- Cookies, cakes, and the like

- Muffins and Croissants

Fats

Selecting fats you consume is also crucial to make a carb cycling diet work. Trans fats and saturated fats are bad. They raise cholesterol in your body, which causes arteries to harden, making you more prone to cardiovascular diseases. Polyunsaturated and monounsaturated fats, on the other hand, are good. They aid in lowering your cholesterol levels, in turn lowering the chances of contracting heart disease. Moreover, they improve the efficiency of insulin.

Good Fat

Here are some foods with good fat.

- Vegetable oil, olive oil, and other plant-based oils – If you'll need oil for cooking, then it's best to use these.

- Avocado

- Sunflower Seeds

- Herring, Mackerel, Trout, Sardines, Tuna, and Salmon, along with other fatty cold-water fish

- Walnuts and Flaxseed

Bad Fat

Here are foods that contain bad fats.

- Animal-based oils

- High-fat dairy products

- Red Meat

- Poultry Skin

- Some vegetable oils (like palm oil and coconut oil)

- French Fries and Potato Chips

- Microwaved Popcorn

- Most Frozen Foods

- Store-bought Baked Goods

- Egg Yolk

Proteins

"Carb" might be in the name of the diet, but proteins can be considered its real "star." Whatever day in the cycle, you got to take in a lot of protein. Proteins build up the muscles, aid in shedding unwanted weight, and keep your tummy full (ergo, keep you from overeating). Moreover, they also serve as building blocks to make your heart, bones, skin, and hair healthy – no matter if you're a bodybuilder or not. Of course, like the two previously discussed nutrients, you must take the right kind of protein. Here are some recommended sources that will fill your protein needs for a carb cycling diet.

- White meat (Poultry) – Poultry meat contains a good deal of protein and little fat. Just take off the skin.

- Milk and other dairy products – Just be careful to choose low-fat variants. They aren't only good sources of protein but also provide calcium.

- Seafood – They are recommended because of their low-fat content. Some fish already mentioned above have higher fat, but they are good fat.

- Soy – High in protein and aids in reducing cholesterol.

- Eggs – One egg a day is good. It has a good amount of protein. Going over that is not a good idea because of the fat.

- Pork Tenderloin – This is another type of white meat and contains lean protein.

- Lean Beef – The fat content is considerably low (comparable to a chicken breast with no skin). It also contains other essential nutrients like vitamin B12, iron, and zinc.

- Beans –They contain a good deal of protein plus they have lots of fiber.

- Protein Powder –They are specially formulated so you can get the right amount of protein efficiently and conveniently.

TOP 5 FACTS ABOUT CARB CYCLING AND FAT LOSS

Carb cycling has become very popular in the world of fat loss simply because it is very effective. It uses a mix of high carb days with low carb days to help you lose weight without needing to starve yourself or experiencing the negative consequences of low carb diet. The negative effects of low carb diet include increased hunger, high craving levels, limited exercise performance, improper metabolism and difficulty in concentrating or focusing at work.

By mixing high carb days with low carb days, you can essentially get rid of the negative effects and lose weight in a more enjoyable way. Following are five facts that you must know before choosing carb cycling.

Heavy Training Should Only Be Done On High Carb Days

The most important thing that you must know about carb cycling is that heavy training should only be done on high carb days. This is because you will require extra energy to carry out heavy workout. This also includes intense cardio. In the absence of sufficient carbs your body will simply not have the energy to carry out heavy gym exercises. And expecting your body to perform normally when it's deprived of the required amount of carbs will only put additional stress on it, which could easily cause muscle damage.

A very important point that you must remember here is that on low carb days the level of glycogen in your body will be low, which means your body's ability to repair or grow muscles will be at its lowest. Therefore, heavy workout on low carb days can cause serious complications. Also, working out hard on high carb days will burn most of your carb intake.

You Will Experience Water Weight Gain

The next thing that you must be prepared for is that you will most likely experience an increase in water weight on high carb days. Your body stores up to 4 g of water for every 1 g of carbohydrate you consume. So if you are consuming approximately 300 g of carbs on high carb days, a significant amount of water will get stored in your body. This is another reason why intense cardio is recommended on high carb days, as it will help you to sweat some water out.

People with leaner body type will experience water weight gain the most, simply because it will be easier to notice it in them. You must not get alarmed because of this. It is part of the process and you are definitely not gaining fat. You will experience an immediate reduction in water weight on low carb days.

Water weight fluctuation can seriously affect people who are psychologically sensitive to weight gain. If you're one of them then you might not enjoy carb cycling as much. However, if you understand the process you will know that this is something that you must deal with in the short term to gain massive long-term benefits.

Carbs Rich in Complex Carbs or Glucose Are Most Beneficial

When it comes to selecting foods that are rich in carbs, your focus must be on glucose. You can select from either simple glucose sources that can be easily used up by the body during workout or complex carbs, which the body can break down into glucose.

Fructose is something you must avoid. This type of carb behaves differently in the body and would not benefit you like glucose does. Enjoying a high fructose meal on a high carb day could still result in weight gain because the body won't be able to store it in the muscles as readily. A good example of high fructose meal is anything that contains high-fructose corn syrup.

Reduce Fat Intake on High Carb Days

There is no doubt in the fact that essential fats are not only good for the body but are also a requirement. However, you must remember to reduce all fat intake apart from essential fats on high carb days to avoid weight gain. Most people think that they can just eat whatever on high carb days and still do good. This is not true at all. The lower you reduce your fat intake on high carb days, the more you will make room for carbohydrates in the body without significantly increasing your calorie intake.

Many people make the common mistake of eating a lot of junk food on high carb days. While junk food is absolutely harmful for the body, it will also make you easily exceed your weekly target for calorie intake.

Maintain Your Target Weekly Calorie Intake Level for Quicker Fat Loss

The final most important fact that you must know about carb cycling is that your weekly intake of calories must not exceed over what is necessary for fat loss. If you do not want to reduce your calorie intake really low on low carb days then you can simply adjust it with the calorie intake on high carb days. This will help you not feel starved on low carb days.

A major mistake that many people make when it comes to carb cycling is that they try to reduce their calorie intake a lot more than required. With carb cycling the expected range of calorie deficit is around 500 to 600 calories, going below that is not only harmful for the body but will also reduce the speed at which you lose weight. For some going below the expected range of calorie deficit could even result in weight gain as the body will go into starvation mode and will try to store as much food as possible as fat within the body.

Balance is the key when it comes to carb cycling. At the end of the day you need to calculate the overall calorie intake during the week and make sure that you don't exceed the required amount.

So there you go, now you have all the information you need to start with carb cycling. You will need a lot of planning, determination and commitment to go through carb cycling. But if you successfully follow it, not only will you lose weight, but will also gain a muscular and healthy body.

LET'S PUT IT TOGETHER

So what exactly does high, low and no carb days look like? You will need to do the math to determine the portion sizes needed based on your weight, but, hopefully, these examples give you an idea of what to look forward to. I will use a 180 pound person so you can also see the numbers you are going for.

High carb day

Here are the guidelines: As many carbs as you want from the approved list at 4/6 or 3/5 of your meals that day. 50-100 calories of fruit at 4/6 or 3/5 meals, 3 cups of non-starchy vegetables or more and 1 gram of protein per pound of body weight divided evenly.

Breakfast: Whole grain English muffin, egg whites (can include one or two yolks), spices, vegetables, serving of fruit

Snack: Protein shake blended with rolled oats

Lunch: Whole grain pasta, chicken, 1 cup vegetables, serving of fruit

Snack: Greek yogurt or protein shake, 1 cup vegetables, serving of fruit

Dinner: Steak, yams, 1 cup vegetables, serving of fruit

Prebed: Small serving tuna, vegetables

If you are eating 5 meals a day simply eliminate the prebed snack and put that amount of vegetables and proteins back into the other meals. You can see also I list more vegetables than recommended, but you can spread them out however you want. If you find a full cup is too much in one sitting, eat a ½ cup 6 times a day. Just do your best to eat three cups a day. Your body will thank you for it.

Low carb day

Here are the guidelines: Same amount of protein and vegetables as high carb day. 1 gram of carbohydrate per pound of body weight from the approved carb list divided over 3/6 or 2/5 meals. 50-100 calories of fruit at 3/6 or 2/5 meals.

Breakfast: Egg Frittata (eggs, mixed vegetables, spices) whole grain toast, serving of fruit

Snack: Protein shake or Greek yogurt or small can tuna

Lunch: Chicken Tortillas with whole grain tortilla, vegetables, salsa, serving of fruit

Snack: Protein shake or Greek yogurt or small can tuna

Dinner: Steak, brown rice, vegetables, serving of fruit

Prebed: Lean protein and vegetables

No carb day

Here are the guidelines: You can basically eat as much protein and vegetables as you want this day. It is also a great day to ensure you consume your healthy fats. You want to feel satisfied during the day to avoid binging or resorting to starchy carbohydrates.

Breakfast: Egg Frittata (eggs, mixed vegetables, spices)

Snack: Protein shake or Greek yogurt or small can tuna

Lunch: Chicken, vegetables, ½ avocado

Snack: Protein shake or Greek yogurt or small can tuna

Dinner: Steak, vegetables

Prebed: Lean protein and vegetables

As you can see, I just removed the carbs from your low carb day to make life easy. If you need to, you can increase your protein go to 1.5 grams per pound of body weight and make sure to include some healthy fats.

Obviously this is just a small sample of what is possible. Even as a weight loss coach knowing what I know, I still check the internet for new recipes, meal combinations or tips on how to make carb cycling easier. Learn how to cook, buy or find some recipe books, and enjoy the food you eat every day.

Breakfast Recipes

Scrambled Eggs with Vegetables

Servings: 2

Nutritional values per serving:

Calories – 338, Fat – 27 g, Carbohydrate – 8 g, Protein – 17 g

Ingredients:

- 4 teaspoons olive oil

- 1 large clove garlic, minced

- 4 large eggs

- ¼ teaspoon salt

- 2 tablespoons cheddar or gouda cheese, shredded

- 1 cup broccoli, chopped

- 1 cup zucchini, chopped

- 1 teaspoon fresh rosemary, minced

- 2 tablespoons heavy cream

- ½ teaspoon pepper powder

Directions:

1. Place a skillet over medium heat. Add oil. When the oil is heated, add broccoli and zucchini and sauté until tender.

2. Add garlic and rosemary and sauté for a few seconds until fragrant.

3. Add eggs, cream, salt, and pepper into a bowl and whisk well. Pour into the skillet. Mix well. Stir frequently until the eggs are nearly cooked.

4. Stir in the cheese and remove the skillet from heat. Mix well.

5. Divide into 2 plates and serve.

Oatmeal with Flax and Chia

Servings: 2

Nutritional values per serving:

Calories – 350, Fat – 14 g, Carbohydrate – 34 g, Protein – 20 g

Ingredients:

- 1 1/3 cups raspberries, divided

- 4 tablespoons chia seeds

- 6 tablespoons flax seed meal

- 1 cup nonfat plain Greek yogurt

- 1 teaspoon vanilla extract

- ½ teaspoon liquid stevia

- 1 cup almond milk, unsweetened

- 1 teaspoon cinnamon powder

Directions:

1. Add half the raspberries into a bowl. Mash with a fork. Add chia seeds, flax seed meal, yogurt, vanilla, stevia, almond milk, and cinnamon. Mix well.

2. Add remaining half of the raspberries and fold gently.

3. Cover and chill for 4-8 hours.

4. Divide into 2 bowls and serve.

Smoked Salmon Breakfast Wraps

Servings: 2

Nutritional values per serving: 1 wrap

Calories – 124, Fat – 6 g, Carbohydrate – 14 g, Protein – 12 g

Ingredients:

- 3 tablespoons light cream cheese spread

- 2 teaspoons lemon zest, finely shredded

- 2 whole wheat flour tortillas (6-7 inches)

- ½ small zucchini, trimmed, peeled into ribbons

- ½ tablespoon fresh snipped chives

- 2 teaspoons lemon juice

- 1.5 ounces smoked salmon, thinly sliced, cut into strips

- Lemon wedges to serve (optional)

Directions:

1. Add cream cheese, lemon juice, lemon zest, and chives into a bowl and stir.

2. Place tortillas on a serving platter. Spread the cream cheese mixture over the tortillas. Do not spread on the edges of the tortillas.

3. Place half the salmon on one-half of the tortillas. Top the salmon with half the zucchini ribbons. Roll from the filled side.

4. Place a wrap in each plate along with a lemon wedge and serve.

Rainbow Frittata

Servings: 2

Nutritional values per serving: 2 wedges

Calories – 219, Fat – 15 g, Carbohydrate – 8 g, Protein – 14 g

Ingredients:

- 1/8 cup sweet potatoes, chopped

- 1/8 cup broccoli, chopped

- ½ teaspoon fresh basil, chopped

- Freshly cracked pepper to taste

- 2 ¾ cups grape or cherry tomatoes, halved

- Nonstick cooking spray

- 1/8 cup yellow bell pepper, chopped

- 4 omega-3 enriched eggs

- ¼ teaspoon snipped fresh thyme

- ½ avocado, peeled, sliced

- Salt to taste

- Sriracha sauce to taste

Directions:

1. Place an ovenproof skillet over medium heat. Spray with cooking spray.

2. When the pan is heated, stir in the bell pepper, sweet potato, and broccoli and sauté until tender. Stir occasionally.

3. Add eggs into a bowl. Whisk well. Add thyme, basil, pepper, and salt and whisk well.

4. Pour into the pan. Do not stir. In a while, the eggs will begin to set. Gently lift the edges with a spatula to allow the raw egg to reach below.

5. Turn off the heat. Place the skillet in a preheated oven.

6. Bake at 400 ° F for about 5-10 minutes or until set.

7. Remove the skillet from the oven and let it rest for a couple of minutes.

8. Cut into 4 equal wedges.

9. Serve 2 wedges in each plate. Top with avocado slices, sriracha sauce, and tomatoes and serve.

Apple Pancakes

Servings: 4

Nutritional values per serving:

Calories – 117, Fat – 6.2 g, Carbohydrate – 14.5 g, Protein – 1.9 g

Ingredients:

- ½ tablespoon broken flax

- 6 tablespoons applesauce

- ½ tablespoon maple syrup

- ½ teaspoon ground cinnamon

- ½ teaspoon baking powder

- 3 tablespoons lukewarm water

- ½ cup oatmeal

- 1 tablespoon coconut oil, melted + extra to fry

- ½ tablespoon vanilla extract

- 1/8 teaspoon salt

Directions:

1. Add broken flax and lukewarm water into a blender and blend until smooth. Let the mixture sit for 10 minutes in the blender.

2. Add applesauce, maple syrup, ground cinnamon, baking powder, lukewarm water, oatmeal, coconut oil, vanilla extract, and salt into the blender. Blend until smooth.

3. If your batter is too thick, add a couple of tablespoons of water and blend again.

4. Pour into a bowl.

5. Place a nonstick pan or griddle over medium heat. Pour about a ¼ cup of the batter. Swirl the pan slightly so that the batter spreads.

6. In a while, bubbles will appear on the pancake, and the edges will begin to get brown. Flip sides and cook the other side until golden brown.

7. Follow steps 5-6 and make the remaining pancakes.

8. Serve warm.

Breakfast Egg White Spinach Enchilada Omelets

Servings: 3

Nutritional values per serving:

Calories – 239, Fat – 12 g, Carbohydrate – 10 g, Protein – 24 g

Ingredients:

- 1 ½ cups egg whites or egg whites from 9 large eggs

- Salt to taste

- Pepper to taste

- ¼ cup scallions + extra to garnish

- A handful fresh cilantro, chopped

- ½ can (from a 4.5-ounce can) chopped green chilies

- ¾ cup low fat Colby Jack cheese, grated

- 1 small avocado, peeled, pitted chopped

- 1 tablespoon water

- Cooking spray

- 1 small ripe tomato, diced

- 5 ounces frozen spinach

- Kosher salt to taste

- Freshly ground pepper to taste

- ½ cup green enchilada sauce

Directions:

1. Take a small baking dish and spread 3 tablespoons enchilada sauce on the bottom of the dish.

2. Add egg whites, salt, pepper and water into a bowl and whisk well.

3. Place a medium-sized nonstick skillet over medium heat. Spray with cooking spray.

4. When the pan is heated, pour about 1/3 of the egg whites into the pan. Swirl the pan so that the whites spread all over the pan. Cook until the omelet is set. Flip sides and cook for 40-60 seconds. Carefully slide on to a plate.

5. Repeat the above 2 steps to make the other 2 omelets.

6. Spray some more cooking spray in the pan. Add scallions and sauté until translucent.

7. Stir in tomato, cilantro, and salt and cook for a couple of minutes.

8. Add spinach and green chili. Sauté for a couple of minutes until the spinach wilts.

9. Add pepper to taste. Turn off the heat. Add ¼ cup cheese and stir.

10. Spread the omelets on your countertop. Divide the mixture among the omelets.

11. Roll and place the omelet rolls in the baking dish, with the seam side facing down.

12. Spread remaining enchilada sauce over the rolls. Sprinkle remaining cheese over the rolls.

13. Cover the baking dish with foil.

14. Bake in a preheated oven at 350 ° F for about 15-20 minutes.

15. Sprinkle scallions and avocado on top and serve.

Lunch Recipes

Classic Falafel

Makes: 12

Nutritional values per serving: 1 falafel without serving options

Calories – 78, Fat – 4 g, Carbohydrate – 8.7 g, Protein – 2.7 g

Ingredients:

- ¾ cup dry chickpeas, rinsed

- ¼ cup white onion, finely chopped

- 1 tablespoon oat flour

- ½ tablespoon cumin powder

- ½ teaspoon coriander powder

- A pinch cardamom powder

- Cayenne pepper to taste (optional)

- ¼ cup fresh parsley, chopped

- 3 cloves garlic, minced

- Salt to taste

- Grape seed oil or any other oil to fry

Directions:

1. Place chickpeas into a pot. Pour enough water to cover the chickpeas by about 2 inches.

2. Place the pot over high heat. When the water begins to boil, let it boil for a couple of minutes. Turn off the heat. Cover and set aside for an hour.

3. Drain and rinse again — Cook the beans in a pressure cooker or instant pot by covering with water. You can also cook in a pot. Cook until soft.

4. Drain and cool the chickpeas. Transfer into a food processor bowl. Process until finely chopped.

5. Add onion, parsley and garlic and pulse until well combined. Add oat flour, cumin, coriander, salt, and cayenne pepper and pulse until well combined. Scrape the sides of the food processor if required.

6. Taste and adjust the salt and spices if necessary. Transfer into a bowl — cover and chill for an hour. If the mixture is very moist, add some more oat flour. If too dry, the process for some more time in the food processor with a sprinkle of water.

7. Divide the mixture into 12 equal portions. Shape into patties.

8. Place a nonstick pan or griddle over medium heat. Add a little oil. Swirl the pan to spread the oil — Fry the falafel in batches.

9. Cook until the underside is golden brown. Flip sides and cook the other side until golden brown.

10. Remove with a slotted spoon and place on a plate lined with paper towels.

11. Serve with pita bread or greens. You can also serve with a low carb dip of your choice.

Parsley and Garlic Chicken Cutlets with Broccoli

Servings: 4

Nutritional values per serving: 12.4 ounces

Calories – 486, Fat – 19 g, Carbohydrate – 15.7 g, Protein – 54 g

Ingredients:

- 8 organic chicken cutlets (about 6-8 ounces each)

- 2 ½ tablespoons olive oil

- 5-6 tablespoons whole wheat pastry flour

- 10 tablespoons dry white wine

- 3 cloves garlic, chopped

- Sea salt to taste

- 1 ½ tablespoons butter, cut into small pieces

- 3 tablespoons fresh parsley, chopped

- 15 ounces fresh broccoli florets

Directions:

1. Place flour in a shallow bowl. Dredge the chicken cutlets in the flour.

2. Place a nonstick skillet over medium-high heat. Add half the oil. When the oil is heated, place a few of the cutlets (cook the remaining in batches). Cook for 3-5 minutes. Flip sides and cook for 3-5 minutes.

3. Meanwhile, add cauliflower into a safe microwave bowl. Microwave on High until tender. It should take 6-7 minutes.

4. Remove the chicken with a slotted spoon and place on a plate lined with paper towels.

5. Add garlic into the same skillet. Sauté until aromatic. Stir in the wine and let it simmer until it is half its original quantity.

6. Remove from heat and stir in the butter, salt, and parsley.

7. Place 2 cutlets in each plate. Pour the butter sauce over it. Place broccoli alongside and serve.

Avocado Ranch Chicken Salad

Servings: 3

Nutritional values per serving: 2/3 cup

Calories – 361, Fat – 23 g, Carbohydrate – 5 g, Protein – 32 g

Ingredients:

- 1 medium ripe avocado, peeled, pitted, scooped

- 1 tablespoon chopped pickled jalapeño

- Salt to taste

- 1 ½ cups shredded or chopped cooked chicken

- 2 tablespoons finely chopped onions

- ¼ cup low carb ranch dressing

- ½ tablespoons white wine vinegar

- Pepper to taste

- ¼ cup celery, chopped

Directions:

1. Add avocado, jalapeño, salt, ranch dressing, vinegar, and pepper into the food processor. Process until smooth. Pour into a bowl.

2. Add chicken, red onion and celery into the bowl and fold gently.

3. Serve as is or chill for a couple of hours and serve later.

Grilled Salmon and Vegetables

Servings: 2

Nutritional values per serving: 1 salmon piece with 1 ¼ cups vegetable

Calories – 281, Fat – 13 g, Carbohydrate – 11 g, Protein – 30 g

Ingredients:

- 1 small zucchini, halved lengthwise

- 1 small red onion, cut into 1-inch wedges

- Salt to taste

- 10 ounces salmon fillets, cut into 2 equal portions

- Lemon wedges to serve

- 1 bell pepper of any color, trimmed, halved, deseeded

- ½ tablespoon extra-virgin olive oil

- Pepper to taste

- A handful of fresh basil, sliced

Directions:

1. Brush a little oil over the onion, bell pepper, and zucchini. Season with salt.

2. Season salmon with salt and pepper.

3. Place all the vegetables and salmon on a preheated grill (place the salmon skin side facing down). Cook the vegetables for 4-6 minutes on each side or until done. Do not turn the salmon while it is cooking. Remove the vegetables and salmon from the grill as it cooks.

4. Place the vegetables on your cutting board. When cool enough to handle, chop into smaller pieces.

5. Place the vegetables in a bowl. Toss well. Discard the skin from the salmon.

6. Serve salmon with vegetables garnished with basil and lemon wedges.

Steak Tacos

Servings: 2

Nutritional values per serving: 2 tacos, without toppings

Calories – 325, Fat – 7 g, Carbohydrate – 29 g, Protein – 37 g

Ingredients:

- Juice of a lime

- ½ teaspoon chili powder

- ¼ teaspoon paprika

- ¼ teaspoon onion powder

- ¼ teaspoon dried oregano

- 4 corn tortillas

- 2 tablespoons chopped onions

- ½ teaspoon salt

- ¼ teaspoon cumin powder

- ¼ teaspoon garlic powder

- Pepper to taste

- 2/3 pound lean sirloin steak, trimmed of fat

- A handful fresh cilantro, chopped

- The ¼ cup of salsa

- ½ tablespoon oil

Directions:

1. Add chili powder, lime juice, paprika, onion powder, oregano, salt, cumin powder, garlic powder, and pepper into a bowl. Mix well.

2. Rub this mixture over the steak.

3. Grill the steak on a preheated grill for 5-6 minutes on each side for medium-rare or the way you like it cooked.

4. When done, place on your cutting board. When cool enough to handle, cut into smaller pieces.

5. Place a skillet over medium heat. Place a skillet over medium heat. Add oil. When the oil is heated, add the chopped steak and sauté for 4-5 minutes.

6. Warm the tortillas following the instructions on the package.

7. Spread the tortillas on your countertop. Place the steak on the tortillas. Garnish with cilantro and any other toppings of your choice if desired. Roll and serve.

Asian Beef Zoodle Soup

Servings: 2

Nutritional values per serving:

Calories –241, Fat – 8.5 g, Carbohydrate – 19.5 g, Protein – 23 g

Ingredients:

- ½ tablespoon coconut oil

- 3 ounces fresh shiitake mushrooms, sliced

- 1 teaspoon fresh ginger, minced

- 1 tablespoon coconut aminos

- ½ teaspoon kosher salt

- 6 ounces beef sirloin steak, boneless, cut into thin slices, across the grain

- ½ small onion, halved, thinly sliced

- 1 clove garlic, minced

- 2 ½ cups beef bone broth

- 1 teaspoon Red Boat fish sauce

- 1 medium zucchini

- For toppings:

- A handful fresh cilantro, chopped

- A handful of fresh basil, chopped

- Lime wedges

- 2 tablespoons thinly sliced green onion

- ½ jalapeño, thinly sliced

Directions:

1. Place a soup pot over medium heat. Add oil. When the oil melts, add onion and sauté until translucent.

2. Stir in the mushrooms and cook for a couple of minutes. Stir in the ginger and garlic and sauté for a few seconds until aromatic.

3. Stir in the broth, fish sauce, coconut aminos, and salt.

4. When it begins to boil, lower the heat to medium low and let it simmer for 4-5 minutes.

5. Meanwhile, make noodles of the zucchini (zoodles) using a spiralizer or a julienne peeler.

6. Add zoodles into the pot and cook for a couple of minutes until slightly tender.

7. Add steak and stir. Let it simmer for a minute.

8. Serve topped with cilantro, basil, green onion, jalapeño, and lemon wedges.

Chicken and Zucchini Burgers

Servings: 8

Nutritional values per serving: Without toppings and bun

Calories – 268, Fat – 13 g, Carbohydrate – 5 g, Protein – 34 g

Ingredients:

- 2 zucchinis, grated

- 1 cup ricotta cheese

- 2 teaspoons garlic powder

- 2 teaspoons kosher salt or to taste

- 1 teaspoon pepper

- 2 pounds 99% lean ground chicken

- 2 eggs

- 2 teaspoons Italian seasoning

- 1 teaspoon onion powder

- 2 tablespoons olive oil

Directions:

1. Place zucchini in a colander. Sprinkle salt and mix. Let it remain in the colander for 10-15 minutes.

2. Squeeze the zucchini of excess moisture using cheesecloth.

3. Place in a bowl. Add ricotta, garlic powder, pepper, chicken, eggs, seasoning and onion powder into the bowl. Mix well. Divide the mixture into 8 equal portions. Shape into burgers.

4. Place a skillet over medium heat. Add half the oil. Place 4 burgers. Cook until the underside is golden brown. Flip sides and cook the other side until golden brown and burger cooked through.

5. Repeat the previous step and cook the remaining burgers.

6. Alternately, you can grill the burgers on a preheated grill.

7. Serve with toppings of your choice or in a low carb bun.

Dinner Recipes

Swedish Meatballs

Servings: 8

Nutritional values per serving: 5 meatballs without noodles

Calories – 213.5, Fat – 10 g, Carbohydrate – 8.5 g, Protein – 25.1 g

Ingredients:

- 2 teaspoons olive oil
- 2 cloves garlic, minced
- ½ cup parsley, minced
- 2 large eggs

- Salt to taste

- Pepper to taste

- 4 cups beef stock

- 2 small onions, minced

- 2 stalks celery, minced

- 2 pounds 93% lean ground beef

- ½ cup seasoned breadcrumbs

- 1 teaspoon ground allspice

- 4 ounces light cream cheese

Directions:

1. Place a skillet over medium heat. Add oil. When the oil is heated, add garlic and onion and sauté until soft.

2. Stir in the parsley and celery and sauté until soft. Turn off the heat and cool for a while. Transfer into a large bowl.

3. Add beef, breadcrumbs, pepper, salt, allspice, and eggs into the bowl of onions. Mix well.

4. Divide the mixture into 40 equal portions and shape into balls.

5. Pour beef stock into the skillet. Place the skillet over medium heat. When it begins to boil, carefully add meatballs into the broth. Cover the skillet with a lid.

6. Carefully remove the meatballs using a slotted spoon and place in a bowl.

7. Pass the stock through a strainer placed over a bowl. Pour the stock into a blender. Add cream cheese and blend until smooth.

8. Pour it back into the skillet. Place the skillet over medium heat. Let the sauce thicken slightly.

9. Pour the sauce into the bowl of meatballs. Stir lightly.

10. Sprinkle parsley and serve as it is or with low carb noodles.

Shrimp Scampi over Zoodles

Servings: 4

Nutritional values per serving: 6 shrimp and ¼ the zoodles

Calories – 170, Fat – 7 g, Carbohydrate – 12 g, Protein – 11 g

Ingredients:

- 4 large zucchinis, trimmed

- 4 teaspoons garlic, minced

- 24 large shrimp, shelled, deveined

- 3 tablespoons fresh lemon juice

- 4 tablespoons low-fat butter or Smart balance light

- ¼ teaspoon crushed red pepper flakes (optional)

- 5 tablespoons white wine or low sodium chicken broth

- 4 teaspoons parmesan cheese, grated

- Salt to taste

- Pepper to taste

Directions:

1. Make noodles of the zucchini (zoodles) using a spiralizer or a julienne peeler.

2. Add zoodles into a microwavable bowl — microwave on High for 2 minutes or until tender.

3. Place a large non-stick pan over medium-low heat. Add butter. When butter melts, add garlic and red pepper flakes and sauté until aromatic. Stir constantly.

4. Stir in the shrimp and sauté until pink. Sprinkle salt and pepper. Remove shrimp with a slotted spoon and place in a bowl.

5. Raise the heat to medium heat. Pour white wine and lemon juice into the pan. Scrape the bottom of the pan to remove any browned bits that may have stuck. Simmer for 2-3 minutes.

6. Stir in the zoodles and shrimp. Mix well. Heat thoroughly.

7. Divide equally the zoodles among 4 plates. Place 6 shrimp on each plate.

8. Sprinkle 1-teaspoon cheese on each plate and serve.

Almond Crusted Pork Tenders

Servings: 8

Nutritional values per serving:

Calories – 293, Fat – 13 g, Carbohydrate – 5 g, Protein – 38 g

Ingredients:

- 2 2/3 pounds lean pork tenderloin, cut into ½ inch thick round slices

- 1 cup almond meal

- 4 teaspoons paprika

- 1 teaspoon salt

- Cooking spray

- 4 egg whites

- ½ cup almonds, sliced

- 1 teaspoon garlic powder

- 1 teaspoon pepper

Directions:

1. Add whites into a wide bowl. Whisk well. Place almond meal, paprika, almonds, salt, garlic powder, and pepper in another wide bowl and stir.

2. First, dip the pork slices in whites. Shake to drop off excess egg. Next dredge in almond meal mixture. Place on a wire rack. Place the wire rack on a baking sheet. Spray cooking spray over the pork on both the sides.

3. Place the baking sheet in the oven.

4. Bake in a preheated oven at 425 ° F for about 15-20 minutes or until cooked through. Broil for the last couple of minutes if you want a crunchy top.

5. Serve.

Turkey Moussaka

Servings: 8

Nutritional values per serving:

Calories – 385, Fat – 16 g, Carbohydrate – 22 g, Protein – 38 g

Ingredients:

- 4 eggplants, cut into ½ inch rounds

- 2 pounds 93% lean ground turkey

- 8 cloves garlic, minced

- 1 cup red wine

- ½ teaspoon ground nutmeg

- ¼ cup parsley, chopped

- 2/3 cup parmesan cheese, grated

- 4 teaspoons extra-virgin olive oil

- 1 large yellow onion, chopped

- 4 tablespoons tomato paste

- ½ teaspoon ground cinnamon

- 24 ounces fat-free Greek yogurt

- 2 eggs

- Salt to taste

- Pepper to taste

Directions:

1. Line a large baking sheet with parchment paper. Spray with cooking spray. Lay the eggplant slices in one layer without overlapping. Roast in batches if required.

2. Spray cooking spray on top of the eggplant slices. Sprinkle salt and pepper.

3. Bake in a preheated oven at 425 ° F for about 5-10 minutes or until light brown. Remove from the oven.

4. Add yogurt, cheese, eggs, half the parsley, salt and pepper into a bowl. Mix well.

5. Place a nonstick skillet over medium-high heat. Add oil. When the oil is heated, add onion and garlic and sauté until soft.

6. Add turkey, salt, and pepper. Sauté until brown.

7. Stir in the nutmeg, cinnamon and tomato paste. Mix until well combined.

8. Pour red wine and stir. Let it cook for 4-5 minutes.

9. Grease a casserole dish with cooking spray. Place eggplant slices on the bottom of the dish. Layer with turkey mixture. Spread it evenly. Spread yogurt mixture evenly on top.

10. Bake in a preheated oven at 425 ° F for about 20 – 30 minutes or until the top is browned as per your liking.

11. Remove from the oven. Cool for a while and serve.

Creamy Cajun Chicken Pasta

Servings: 8

Nutritional values per serving: 2 cups

Calories – 344, Fat – 10 g, Carbohydrate – 23 g, Protein – 37 g

Ingredients:

- 2 spaghetti squashes, halved, deseeded

- 4 tablespoons Cajun seasoning, divided or more to taste

- 2 green bell peppers, thinly sliced

- 2 red bell peppers, thinly sliced

- 1 red onion, thinly sliced

- 2 cans (14 ounces each) fire-roasted diced tomatoes with its liquid

- ½ cup scallions

- 2 2/3 pounds chicken breast, skinless, boneless, chopped into chunks

- 4 teaspoons olive oil

- 4-6 cloves garlic, minced

- 1 cup low fat cream cheese

Directions:

1. Spray the cut part of the spaghetti squash halves with cooking spray. Cover each of the squash halves with foil. Place the squash halves on a baking sheet.

2. Bake in a preheated oven at 375 ° F for about 45-60 minutes or until tender.

3. When done, unwrap and cool for a while. When cool enough to handle, scrape the flesh of the squash with a fork. Place in a bowl discards the outer covering of the squash.

4. Place chicken in a bowl. Sprinkle half the Cajun seasoning over the chicken and toss well. Place a large skillet over medium heat. Add oil. When the oil is heated, add chicken. Sauté until tender.

5. Add bell peppers and onion and sauté for 3-4 minutes.

6. Lower the heat to low heat. Stir in the tomatoes, half the Cajun seasoning, and cream cheese.

7. When the cream cheese melts, turn off the heat. Taste and adjust salt and pepper if required.

8. Add chicken and shredded spaghetti squash. Toss well.

9. Garnish with scallions and serve.

Thai Green Curry

Servings: 4

Nutritional values per serving: Without rice

Calories – 380, Fat – 32.4 g, Carbohydrate – 18.5 g, Protein – 9.4 g

Ingredients:

- For the green curry:

- 1 sweet potato, peeled, cut into cubes

- 1 ½ cups broccoli florets

- 1 ½ can (14 ounces each) coconut milk

- 2 teaspoons olive oil

- Salt to taste

- 2 tablespoons Thai green curry paste

- 24 ounces firm tofu

- Optional:

- 1 tablespoon golden raisins

- A handful fresh cilantro, chopped

- A dash of fish sauce

- Brown sugar to taste

- Cooked rice

Directions:

1. Press the tofu of excess moisture using paper towels. Chop into cubes.

2. Place a soup pot over medium-high heat. Add oil. When the oil is heated, add tofu and salt and sauté until brown. Remove tofu with a slotted spoon and set aside.

3. Place the pot back over heat. Add coconut milk and curry paste and stir until well combined. Add sweet potatoes and cook until tender.

4. Stir in the broccoli and tofu cook for 3-4 minutes or until broccoli is crisp as well as tender.

5. Add the optional ingredients if using and stir.

6. Serve with rice.

CONCLUSION

Thanks for purchasing this book. It's my firm belief that it has provided you with all the answers to your questions.

With all of this information, you now have the knowledge you need to start carb cycling and working out to reach your health and fitness goals. Hopefully, you also have the motivation to make the first moves on your journey. Carb cycling is a flexible way to eat healthfully while not depriving yourself. Carb cycling based on your fitness activities will help you to reach your health and fitness goals in a realistic and safe way. Make it work for you, and you will find benefits for your physical and mental wellbeing, and you can begin to show others the way as well. Remember that you are not alone in this journey – carb cycling together with appropriate exercising is a route now taken by more and more people – if you need it you can find case study blogs online or in books – this might help you get started, but remember that the longest journeys begin with one step – this relates to diet just as much as exercise.

The information in this guide is designed as a base – the beauty of carb cycling is that it can be customized to your needs. If you need them, there are many more resources available to help you get started on your health and fitness journey. You can consult with doctors, nutritionists, and physical trainers. You can search online for websites, blogs, and databases. There is also a great deal of YouTube videos that aim to help people reach their goals. You can read books to learn more about nutrition and whole natural foods, or maybe you could drop into that wholefood shop you pass from time to time. The point is you have the power to make informed choices as to what to do next.

While all these back-up information sources and support mechanisms are very important, it is also important to remember that you are already beginning to make the first steps by yourself. By beginning to think through alternative ways of eating or exercising, you are empowering yourself to take decisions which can help you to reach your long terms goals.

With the information you have just read, as well as the other information available to you, there is really nothing holding you back from creating a new way of eating and working out to help you to reach your goals. The only thing that can keep you from your goals now is you, so get out there, clear your head and then start making a plan for how you intend to reach your goals. The next step is to create a weekly meal and exercise plan and stick to it for a week. Monitor your progress and see if you can extend the plan to a month. Don't forget your reward days – but don't make them every day! If you find your plan is really not working out the way you had hoped, then it is not a lost cause - consult all of your resources again and alter your plan until you find what works best for you. Go for it, stick to it, and reap the benefits. You can do this, and who knows, maybe you will be the inspiration to others around you to make similar positive changes in their lives.

What is most important is that the changes you make result in clear benefits to you. By trying to find information on how to make lifestyle changes and learn more about the choices available, you have already begun the journey. By now understanding the options available, you are well placed to begin to make informed choices – remembering that you are allowed reward days. What happens next is entirely up to you – it is you that is in control!